Is Your Environment Stressing You Out?

How to Pro-Actively Protect Yourself From Environmental Toxins

Dr. Kelly Miller, DC, NMD, FASA, FBAARM, CFMP

Is Your Environment Stressing You Out?
How to Pro-Actively Protect Yourself From Environmental Toxins

Book 3 of the *Health Restoration Series*
Series Editor, George Ann Gregory, Ph.D.

Printed by CreateSpace, An Amazon.com Company
CreateSpace, Charleston, SC

ISBN 13: 978-0-9979113-6-7
ISBN 10: 0997911336

Dedication

I dedicate this book to all the people who are seeking information about how to stay healthy in an environmentally challenged world.

Acknowledgement

I could not have written this book without the support and encouragement of my best friend and soul mate, Dr. Debra Hoffman. I would like to give a special thanks to Genova Diagnostics, Great Plains Laboratory, Inc, Oxford Laboratory, Vollara™, and Multipure™ for giving me liberal use of their information in printed format and from the Internet. I give thanks to my sister, Dr. George Ann Gregory for her editing, and Emz Wright for the book cover.

I have been guided by the following Biblical passages.

Proverbs 8:1-36, 9:1

Does wisdom not cry out, and understanding lift up her voice? She takes her stand on the top of the high hill, beside the way, where the paths meet. She cries out by the gates, at the entry of the city, at the entrance of the doors: "To you, O men, I call, and my voice is to the sons of men. O you simple ones, understand prudence, and you fools, be of understanding heart. Listen, for I will speak of excellent things, and from the opening of my lips, will come right things. For my mouth will speak truth: wickedness is an abomination to my lips. All the words of my mouth are with righteousness; nothing crooked or perverse is in them. They are all plain to him that understands, and right to those who find knowledge. Receive my instruction, and not silver, and knowledge rather than choice gold; For wisdom is better than rubies, and all the things one may desire cannot be compared to her. "I, wisdom, dwell with prudence, and find out knowledge and discretion. The fear of the Lord is to hate evil; pride and arrogance and the evil way and perverse mouth I hate. Counsel is mine, and sound wisdom; I am understanding, I have strength. By me kings reign, and rulers decree justice. By me princes rule, and nobles, all the judges of the earth. I love those who love me, and those who seek me diligently will find me. Riches and honor are with me, enduring riches and righteousness. My fruit is better than gold, yes, than fine gold, and my revenue than fine silver. I transverse the way of righteousness, in the midst of justice, That I may cause those who love me to inherit wealth, that I may fill their treasures. "The Lord possessed me, at the beginning of His way, before His works of old. I have been established from everlasting.

From the beginning, before there was an earth. When there was no depth I was brought forth, when there were no fountains abounding with water. Before the mountains were settled, before the hills, I was brought forth; while as yet He had not made the earth or the fields, or the primal dust of the world. When He prepared the heavens, I was there, when He drew a circle on the face of the deep, When He established clouds above, when He strengthened the fountains of the deep, When He assigned to the sea its limit, so that the waters would not transgress His command, when He marked out the foundations of the earth, Then I was beside Him as a master craftsman; and I was daily His delight, rejoicing always before Him, Rejoicing in His inhabited world, and my delight was with the sons of men. "Now therefore, listen to me my children, for blessed are those who keep my ways. Hear instruction and be wise, and do not disdain it. Blessed is the man who listens to me, watching daily at my gates, waiting at the posts of my doors. For whoever finds me finds life, and obtains favor from the Lord; But he who sins against me wrongs his own soul; all those who hate me love death." Wisdom has built her house, she has hewn out her seven pillars. *NKJV*

Proverbs 9:9-11
Give instruction to a wise man, he will be yet wiser: teach a just man, and he will increase in learning. For the fear of the Lord is the beginning of wisdom; and the knowledge of the holy is understanding. For by me thy days shall be multiplied and the years of thy life shall be increased. *NKJV*

James: 13-17
Who is wise and understanding among you? Let him show by good conduct that his works are done in the meekness of wisdom. But if you have bitter envy and self-seeking in your hearts, do not trust and lie against the truth. This wisdom does not descend from above, but is earthly, sensual, demonic. For where envy and self-seeking exist, confusion and every evil thing are there. But the wisdom that is from above is first pure, then peaceable, gentle, willing to yield, full of mercy and good fruits, without partiality and without hypocrisy. *NKJV*

Disclaimer

This publication is designed to provide scientific, authoritative, and personal anecdotal information in regard to the subject matter covered. The reader understands that the author is not engaged in rendering professional services. If you require medical, psychological, or any other expert assistance, please seek the services of a professional.

The information, personal experiences, anecdotal stories, procedures, and suggestions contained in the book are not intended to replace the services of a trained health-care professional or to serve as a replacement for a health-care professional's advice and care. You should consult a health-care professional regarding any of this information, ideas, personal experiences, anecdotal stories, procedures, supplements, drug therapies, or any other information from this book.

The author hereby specifically disclaims any and all liability arising directly or indirectly from the use or application of any of the products, ideas, procedures, drug therapies, or suggestions contained in this book and any errors, omissions, and inaccuracies in the information contained herein. The treatments and supplements included in this book are for identification purposes only and are not intended to recommend or endorse the product.

Preface

I discovered the importance of nutrition in 1978 at the age of 22 when my senior clinician at chiropractic school recommended I stop drinking milk and start taking betaine HCL with my meals. I was amazed and pleasantly surprised to find my digestive dysfunction and reoccurring urinary tract infections went away and never returned. One of my early mentors was Dr. M.T. Morter, Jr., who was president of Logan University while I attended and later authored several books. He was a proponent of alkalizing the body with foods and supplements that contained potassium, magnesium, zinc, selenium, and the like. One of the supplements I recommended in those days for my patients was *Green Magma,* a green powder made from barley sprouts, because of its mineral content. Generally speaking, the patient population of the late seventies and early eighties was much healthier than the patients of today and needed less supplementation than the patients of today.

It has been known for some time that there have been significant mineral and vitamin deficiencies in the soil and the food sources in the United States for over eighty years. I found an interesting article from *Cosmopolitan* magazine concerning a report from Congress in 1936 about this mineral loss in the soil and foods in the U.S. Things have not gotten better since 1936, but have become worse, much worse. Compounding the nutritional deficiencies in modern diets since WWII is the introduction of some 80,000 plus environmental chemicals. It is not a question if you have a nutritional deficiency—you do. It is more of a question of how many and how severe the deficiencies are.

Today, we have the technology not only to evaluate specific vitamin, mineral, amino acids, fatty acids, and anti-oxidants in individuals, but to also assess and quantify the body burden (toxicity levels) of specific environmental toxins consumed via drinking water, air, and foods. In addition to the obvious need to eliminate as many sources of these toxins as possible, you also need supplementation of specific nutrients to aid in detoxification of the body.

This book builds on the data presented in Book 1, *13 Secrets of Optimal Aging,* and Book 2, *Micronutrient Testing.* If you have not yet read the first 2 books in this series, I recommend that you do.

—

Table of contents

Introduction

This is my third book in the Health Restoration series. If you missed the first two, they are *13 Secrets to Optimal Health: How Your Hormones Can Help You Achieve a Better Quality of Life and Longevity* and *Micronutrient Testing: How to Find What Vitamins, Minerals, and Antioxidants You Need.* Each book in the series compliments each other and gives additional information about the nine variables to good health—genetic variants, environmental toxins, trauma, what we eat, what we drink, how we exercise, how we rest, how/what we breathe, and what we think. What we think is the most important because it determines our choices, lifestyle, and behavior. The purpose of this book is to increase your awareness about potential causes of your illness (a chronic dysfunction like fatigue or lack of energy without any named source)/disease (named condition) from environmental toxins so you can make better decisions concerning your health and well-being. This potential causation for less than optimal health may not even be on your or your doctors' radar. If you don't know what the environmental causes of disease are, you cannot test for it or correct it.

This book, like the previous two, discusses signs, symptoms, illnesses, and diseases that can be verified by specific testing and corrected by changes in lifestyle and specific supplementation. If you are reading this, you are open to the possibility that environmental toxicity may be the cause or contributing factor of your health problems or those of a close friend or relative. This is the correct perception to have. It is not a question of whether or not you have environmental toxins in your body: You do. It is a matter of how many toxins there are and the quantity of each. I have never had a patient who was evaluated that did not have significant levels of several different dangerous chemicals in their bodies. Many of you may be wondering how many environmental toxins are in your body. It is probably much more than you have imagined. Although there are studies that involve the effects of a single environmental pollutant, I have not found any that study the cumulative effects of multiple toxins. However, I think it is logical to assume that having high levels of several environmental toxins is more dangerous than having a single toxin. At the end of the book, there are case histories that will give you an idea of what kind of conditions exposure to these toxins can cause, how their presence is demonstrated and the amount of each (*body burden*), and how to reduce and eliminate these from the body.

The Seven Sequela of Stress

One of the points made in my first book, *13 Secrets to Optimal Aging*, is that all stressors cause a fight/flight response accompanied by an increase in adrenaline followed by a corresponding increase in cortisol. This causes a shift in the balance of the autonomic nervous system with the sympathetic nervous system dominating, which is the first consequence or *sequela* of stress. The stressor causing the fight/flight response can be the result of many different situations, for example, a house fire; being robbed at gunpoint; a pending attack of a hundred-pound Rottweiler; any worry, fear, or apprehension; physical trauma from a fall, sports-related injury, car crash, or running a marathon; sleep deprivation; eating excess trans-fats or high fructose corn syrup; drinking too much alcohol, sodas, or even fruit juice. All of these stressors decrease hormone levels over time, thus creating the second sequala of stress.

Hormone levels are a gauge of how well an individual is doing relative to the potential stress of the 9 variables—genetic variances, environmental toxins, trauma, diet (food and drink), amount of rest, amount of exercise, breathing environment (how and what), and thoughts. These factors determine each individual's hormone levels, relative health and well-being. Environmental toxins are a stressor that subsequently adversely affects hormone levels.

The third sequela to stress is nutritional deficiencies, one of the points made in my second book *Micronutrient Testing*. Specifically, certain micronutrients are depleted in an attempt to detoxify and eliminate environmental toxins. For example, in order to eliminate mercury, the body consumes magnesium, selenium, and glutathione in an attempt to chelate (bind), detoxify, and subsequently eliminate the mercury.

The fourth sequela of stress caused by environmental toxins is the thickening and stickiness of the platelets and red blood cells result from stressor. In the 1980s, dark field microscopy was popular for observing this phenomenon. At this time, I made the observation that all kinds of stressors can cause this clumping of platelets and red blood cells since this is a common response to any stressor causing inflammation. I also observed that different chemicals and conditions—including, but not limited to, aspirin, omega-3, B6, Vitamin D, magnesium, changes in electrical or electromagnetic energy, listening to music of a certain frequency, or dramatic positive mental or spiritual changes—may cause de-clumping or reduction of the stickiness of the platelets and red blood cells. As all stressors, including environmental toxins, cause inflammation and inflammation causes clumping of the platelets and red blood cells, it is easy to understand the proliferation of allopathic physician prescribed anti-inflammatories and herbs like *turmeric* and *boswellia* recommended by chiropractors and naturopathic physicians.

The fifth sequela of stress is environmentally caused damage to the endothelium. Chronic stressors producing inflammation adversely affect the *glycocalyx*, a Teflon-like coating that covers the surface of the endothelium, that single-celled layer of cells that protects the blood vessels and forms the brain blood barrier through tight junctions. The glyocalyx is something you will be hearing and reading more about as time goes by. It appears to be a key in protecting the endothelium from trauma, oxidation, and plaquing. Stressors—trans-fats, sugar, alcohol, mercury, worry, and the like—adversely affect the glyocalyx, which in turn allows the endothelium to be injured. This injury results in oxidation, plaquing, and calcification. All these factors influence the elasticity of the blood vessel, the ability of the blood vessels to dilate or expand. All these factors not only make the platelets and red blood cells clump together, thereby making them more difficult to pass through the smaller blood vessels, but they also the influence the ability of the blood vessel to dilate to allow more blood flow to the tissues. The persistence of these two simultaneous responses for too long a period of time undermine the health of the individual by reducing blood flow that carries oxygen and micronutrients to the tissues.

The sixth sequela of stress is decrease in the amount of protective *SIgA* (*Secretory IgA*) and a loosening of the tight junctions causing hyperpermeability, aka, *leaky gut*. Environmental toxins can cause inflammation, leaky gut, and an autoimmune-like response. Chronic stress and inflammation also adversely affects the SIgA, the mucous membrane that protects the GI tract and the source of much of acquired immunity. Prolonged cumulative stressors that cause inflammation thin the SIgA. The decrease in SIgA production and function occurs as both cortisol and DHEA hormone levels become low. This also influences a loosening of the *tight junctions* in the epithelium of the small intestine. The epithelium consists of the single cell layer of cells that provides protection by selectively allowing nutrients to be absorbed and passed into the rest of the body. This loosening causes increased inflammatory responses from the body involving white blood cells that can lead to an over-sensitized immune system and an auto-immune-like response. This loosening allows change in the natural microbiome environment as well.

The seventh sequela of stress is damage to the *mRNA* (messenger RNA), which holds the transcription or duplication information of the mitochondria. Mitochondria are very susceptible to damage. Superoxide dismutase is the anti-oxidant that protects the mitochondrial membrane. As this compound becomes deficient, the mitochondria become susceptible to infiltration, damaging the mRNA. As a result, an increased number of mitochondria become less efficient in producing cellular energy. Environmental toxins cause inflammation that can cause mitochondrial dysfunction. Mitochondrial dysfunction is now recognized as being involved with all chronic illness/disease. Organs particularly susceptible to develop symptoms are the heart, liver, and brain as they have the greatest number of mitochondria.

The seven sequela of stress—autonomic imbalance, hormone deficiencies, micronutrient deficiencies, blood/platelet stickiness, inhibition of the glycocalyx/endothelium damage, depletion of Secretory IgA/loosening of tight junctions/change in microbiome, and mRNA/mitochondria damage— are a commonality in all chronic diseases.

One of the many problems in our health care system in the U.S. (I call it our health crisis management system) is there is so much specialization that the doctor of the specialty—gastroenterology, urology, cardiovascular, and the like—only looks at that single organ or organ systems. Most allopathic physicians only treat symptomatically one area with a pharmaceutical agent that often has an adverse effect on another organ or organ system. These medical practitioners often miss the big picture and the root cause of the problem because they are only looking at a few of the symptoms of the cumulative effects of stress (inflammation). As a consequence, they may treat the part to the detriment of the whole. These modern practitioners have lost the necessary skills of listening to a patient's history, asking him/her the right questions, and observing the patient—eyes, hair, skin, size, shape, smell, and the like. The art of consultation and the physical exam has been lost by many and replaced with a battery of tests. I am telling you now that allopathic medicine is headed in the direction of computer diagnosis and prescription of medication that will outperform the current system of doctor diagnosis and prescription. This, however, is not the type of practice I promote.

In a modern urban setting, the fight/flight response, triggering the adrenal glands, works overtime. Hans Selye, a Nobel Prize winner, described The General Adaptive Syndrome, involving the adrenal glands in a stress response, in three phases: alarm, reactive, and exhaustion. It wasn't until my education as a Fellow in the Brazil-American Aging and Regenerative Medicine and my Certification in Functional Diagnostic Medicine that I began to more fully appreciate the hormonal influence/reaction to stress. In the fight/flight response, adrenaline production rapidly occurs. The adrenaline (epinephrine) is produced in the adrenal medulla. The effects of adrenaline are multiple.

- It activates the body fat into fatty acids to provide instant energy to the mitochondria of the cells.
- It contracts the pupils for sharper vision.
- It increases the heart rate and blood flow to the big skeletal muscles for maximum power.

This physiological response aids us to fight off the tiger or run away like a world-class sprinter. Shortly after this adrenaline response, another part of the adrenal gland, called the cortex, produces cortisol. Cortisol is a glucocorticoid that facilitates the production of glucose. By design, the extra glucose can help sustain energy needed for the emergency or to help repair the injured tissues from the fight or flight that just occurred, and it is a powerful anti-inflammatory. This mechanism was designed to occur every once in a while, not continually. This fight/flight response occurs with both real and imagined dangers. Sensational news reports increase a sense of danger for many people. This phenomenon is so common that some mental health practitioners have suggested that people forgo reading or listening to the news.

Because of the current much-too-complicated and polluted world, this fight/flight response occurs 24/7 for many of us. In *13 Secrets to Optimal Aging,* I presented the concept of a prolonged stress response and the problems it caused in a diagram called pregnenolone steal. Although it is a bit more complicated than this, this diagram demonstrates what happens to the endocrine (hormone) system when a person experiences on-going stress. The majority of the hormone production becomes shunted into cortisol, causing a decrease in the production of anabolic (tissue-building) hormones like DHEA, testosterone, and estradiol. See the pregnenolone steal diagram below.

Pregnenolone Steal
The Adverse effects of Stress
© Kelly Miller, DC NMD FASA FBAARM

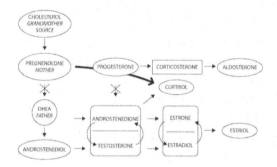

The idea is that, for many, their environment causes a never-ending fight/flight response. Stressors have a cumulative effect throughout a lifetime, which results in an inability to maintain homeostasis. It is little wonder so many are so ill. Specifically, the water we drink, shower and bathe in, and swim in along with the air we breathe at home and/or work and the toxin-laden food we eat relentlessly attacks our bodies, breaking down the immune and detoxification systems. A prolonged fight/flight response leads to inflammation with subsequent hormone depletion, micronutrient depletion, sticky blood, endothelial vascular damage, small intestine hyperpermeability (leaky gut), and mitochondrial dysfunction. In order to get healthier, you need to eliminate, or at least greatly reduce, the burden of heavy metals, pesticides, herbicides, petroleum byproducts, PBAs, PCBs, and the like in the body.

This book, the third in a seven-book series called *Health Restoration*, reveals potential causes for chronic illness and diseases that most individuals and doctors have not considered. For example, mercury toxicity can cause two common health problems— hypertension and hypothyroidism. Assessing the hypertensive or hypothyroid patient for mercury toxicity is not even on the radar for most physicians. The average allopathic doctor will prescribe an ACE inhibitor, beta-blocker, calcium channel blocker, or a diuretic for hypertension without looking for any specific causation. In general, most hypertension is not well managed and many patients are placed on a cocktail of multiple different drugs in an attempt to keep the blood pressure under control.

The root cause of the hypertension could be from an environmental toxin such as mercury or a nutritional deficiency of magnesium, coenzyme Q10, Vitamin D, Vitamin K2, B vitamins, or something else. By the way, if a prescription calcium channel blocker is effective, magnesium will work just as well. If an ACE inhibitor works, so will glutathione. A person does not become ill because s/he has drug deficiencies, but a person can and does often suffer from vitamin, mineral, fatty acid, and anti-oxidant deficiencies. Drugs are great for emergencies where they save lives, but they are not great for chronic health conditions. It is not the allopathic doctor's fault s/he doesn't know any of this. They are doing the best they can, based upon their education, which is largely controlled by the pharmaceutical manufacturers. Any practitioner who has seen patients for over thirty years has observed an ever-growing population of younger patients suffering from chronic disease that used to only occur in a smaller population of the elderly.

In the case of hypothyroidism, the TSH (thyroid-stimulating hormone) is used for screening. One of the many problems with this reference range is that it much too broad, having a reference range of 1000 percent. New evidence indicates this test only picks up about 18 % of the people suffering from hypothyroidism. In 1980 when I became a physician, a standard thyroid screening consisted of not only TSH, but also T4, and T3 levels as well. Somewhere along the line, doctors became convinced they did not need to assess these values. Even with testing T4 and T3 levels, many patients are missed because of T3 receptor resistance. It is the T3 that is the bioactive form of the hormone that drives the cellular metabolism. It is not the amount of free T3 that is available in the serum that is the key. Rather, it is how much T3 that gets inside the cell via the cell membrane receptors that is important. Unfortunately for you as the patient, this is something most doctors do not understand. Reverse T3 (rT3) or high levels of cortisol or environmental toxins can inhibit loss of T3 sensitivity. Most doctors prescribe either Synthroid or levothyroxine, which are synthetic forms of T4 for the hypothyroid condition. Approximately half of these patients still remain symptomatic after medication. The physicians mistakenly assume that a person will be able to convert the T4 to T3. As long as the TSH is in reference range, they look no further, despite the patient's symptomatology remaining unchanged. Health is more than a number on a lab test. The question of whether the thyroid is not working due to an excess body burden of mercury or another toxin like arsenic, chloride, fluoride, bromine, or perhaps excess PCBs or PBAs from the environment is never asked. Perhaps the condition is caused because of an iodine, selenium, zinc, or Vitamin D deficiency.

Most allopathic physicians look no further than the TSH. If any of the environmental toxins or nutritional deficiencies are the cause, sooner or later there will be more organs affected unless the underlying cause of the condition is corrected. It is better to find the root cause and correct it immediately. Otherwise, a physician is only symptom chasing, and worse problems will have to be dealt with later.

In 2005, the Environmental Working Group conducted an interesting study on ten Americans. The blood analysis consisted of analyzing 413 different chemicals, including heavy metals, PBAs, PCBs, chlorinated pesticides, herbicides, and there were 287 different chemicals found in these ten individuals with each individual averaging over 200 distinct toxic environmental chemicals. The results of the analysis were quite remarkable. Twenty-eight chemicals were waste byproducts coming from incinerator and smoke stacks. Forty-seven were consumer products, such as flame-retardants, pesticides, herbicides, and the like. The most disturbing finding was that there were 212 different industrial chemicals that had been banned for over 30 years.

This study was the first time since the introduction of all these chemicals into the environment that anyone had done an analysis on the blood in the umbilical cord.

- One hundred and thirty-four (134) chemicals in the umbilical cord have been found to cause cancer in laboratory studies or in animals.
- One hundred and fifty-one (151) chemicals have been found to be associated with birth defects. One hundred and fifty-eight chemicals, like lead, mercury, and PCBs, were neurotoxins that cause profound adverse effects on intelligence, behavioral development, and motor coordination.
- One hundred and fifty-four (154) chemicals are known endocrine (hormone) disrupters, adversely affecting hypothalamus, pituitary, thyroid, or gonadal function.
- One hundred and eighty-six (186) chemicals cause infertility.
- One hundred and thirty (130) chemicals are toxic to the immune system.

As you can see, many of these chemicals have multiple adverse consequences on the future development and function of the fetus. In fact, a 2006 article published in *Lancet* stated that the combined evidence suggests that neurodevelopmental disorders resulting from industrial chemicals has caused a silent pandemic in our modern society.[1]

It is alarming that these chemicals were in the mother's blood that was assigned to encourage the growing fetus. About three hundred quarts of blood are circulated to the developing fetus every day. A significant fact is that a developing fetus has no blood brain barrier protection, so the developing brain has no protection from any chemicals as it will after a couple of years. It has been believed that the placenta was able to filter out these toxins. Sadly, this is not the case, so unfortunately environmental toxin exposure begins in the womb. The presence of these chemicals does not mean necessarily that biological damage does occur to the fetus. However, their presence should raise concern because the chemicals put a tremendous stress on a very young and developing detoxification and anti-oxidation systems in the fetus and infant.

The presence of these toxins cause nutrients like glutathione, selenium, zinc, calcium, magnesium, and B Vitamins, such as riboflavin, folate, B6, B12, niacin, and thiamine, to be used up at a higher rate in an attempt to rid toxins from the body. In fact, any nutrient that is used in the mitochondrial energy chain production has the potential of being depleted due to increased detoxification clearance for the fetus or infant. If the increased exposure is coupled with a poor dietary intake by the mother, the depleted vitamin/mineral soil content renders fewer vitamins, minerals, and antioxidants in the mother's blood supply to the developing fetus. Failure of the detoxification and anti-oxidation systems ensues. These consequences are why a good diet, natural vitamin/mineral/anti-oxidant pre-natal and nursing formulae, a pure water source, and pure air are so critical to the proper development of fetuses and infants. Inadequate micronutrient levels in the mother greatly increase the potential negative effects of the environmental toxins. Proactive measures should be taken to greatly reduce or eliminate the environmental toxins from the mother's body. (There will be additional information in *How to Have a Healthy Baby and Child in Today's World*, a future publication.)

Each year, there are a higher percentage of children diagnosed with attention deficit hyperactivity disorder (ADHD) and autism. The CDC estimates that 1 in 25 children may soon be at risk for autism spectrum syndrome. The incidence of autism had been 1 in 10,000 for three decades before the increased schedule of vaccines containing mercury for children was adopted. In 1983, most children had ten recommended vaccinations by age six. After 2013, 36 vaccinations have been recommended by age six. No intellectually honest physician can say that the children of today are healthier than they were 30 plus years ago. More recently, many vaccines have been switched from mercury to aluminum as a preservative. Aluminum, like mercury, is also a neurotoxin. Some vaccines contain both mercury and aluminum, which exponentially increases the risk of brain/nervous system injury. The levels of mercury and aluminum exceed the safe limits set by the EPA for adults through ingestion via the GI tract, yet infants and small children are given these doses directly into the bloodstream. Most people don't realize that they are getting potential mercury poisoning with every tetanus and flu shot.

Additionally, over the last 20 years, the number of allergies and asthma cases has tripled with fifty million Americans now suffering with one or the other. Another 50 million Americans have some form of auto-immune-like illness/disease. In 1930, only 1 person in 3,000 was diagnosed with cancer. Today, 1 in 3 women and 1 in 2 men will likely be diagnosed with cancer in their lifetime. This is a frightening state of affairs and should be a wake-up call to all of us. Each of us, as individuals, must take personal responsibility for our own health and the health of our loved ones.

Despite the obvious questions, the chemical industry, of course, say their chemicals are safe because these chemicals only exist in a few ppb (parts per billion). The industry further questions how such a minute amount causes any problems. It is interesting to note that most prescription drugs themselves are active at only a few ppb. Here are a few examples. Albuterol, a drug used every day by many asthmatics and probably in every school nurse's medicine cabinet is effective at 2.1 ppb. Paxil, a commonly used antidepressant that you have probably seen advertised on television is active at a dose of 30 ppb. Cialis, a medication advertised for erectile dysfunction that works up to 36 hours, is effective at a level of 30 ppb. Nuvaring, a contraceptive medication, is effective at a dose of only 0.0035 ppb. Even at these low doses, individuals often suffer severe side effects due to genetic variants and nutritional deficiencies that influence an individual's ability to metabolize any given substance. Even minute amounts of certain substances can have profound negative side effects on a susceptible individual.

The presence of these minute amounts of only a few ppb has a significant negative impact on the U.S. population as the presence of medications has been detected in many city municipality water systems. An Associated Press study involving one city in all 50 different states discovered the presence of multiple medications in the water supply of about 41million Americans. The medications came from the urine and feces of people taking the medications as well as the occasional flush of an out-of-date prescription. None of these cities are attempting to clean up the water.[2]

These minute quantities become a problem because most of these toxins accumulate in the body, generally stored in body fat with some like lead being stored in the bone. These environmental toxins are accumulated by a woman during pregnancy and passed through to the fetus. Accumulations of small amounts of environmental toxins may affect fertility. For example, 20% of American couples have problems with conception. The largest portion of the problem has been in women who are under twenty-five years of age. The sperm count of men in the United States and Northern Europe has been declining by 1% each year for the past 25 years. The Massachusetts Study on Men, the largest ongoing epidemiological study of men's testosterone levels, shows a steady decline in testosterone over the past 30 years.

Genetics alone does not explain an increased incidence of many conditions in children. Between 1975 and 2002, there was an 84% increase in acute lymphocytic anemia in children. The incidence of hypospadius, a birth defect causing the urethra to emerge somewhere besides the end of the penis, has doubled in the last 20 years. Now, 1 baby boy in every 125 is born with this condition, requiring surgery within days or weeks of birth. Certain chemicals are associated with this effect. There has been a 57% increase in childhood brain cancers. An increase in cancer is just not confined to children. Breast cancer now occurs in 1 in 8 women in the United States. By this time, you may be feeling overwhelmed with the information and are wondering what can be done about all these exposures. In the chapters to follow, I discuss the potential problems with certain chemicals, the source of these chemicals, and solutions to avoid or correct illnesses and diseases that can result from these exposures.

Reference List
1. Grandjean P, Landrigan P. *Lancet: chemical exposure creating a "silent pandemic" of neurodevelopmental disorders?* http://www.medscape.com/viewarticle/...4005&src=nldne. Published November 8, 2006. Accessed Nov 28, 2017.
2. MSNBC. *Drugs in water.* https://youtu.be/--c8BtASRJ4. Published Jan 3, 2016. Accessed Nov 28, 2017.

Chapter 1: Some of Today's Health Challenges

Patients today do not respond as well to treatment as they did in the past. It was much easier to get patients well in 1980 than today. Most patients today are locked into a sympathetic dominance (fight/flight response). This is based on my experience of performing hundreds of heart rate variability tests on my patients. Heart rate variability measures the time between heartbeats. Although most of us think a steady heart beat is good, nothing could be further from the truth. The fact is the less variance a person has in his/her heartbeat the more likely the person will be chronically ill and die. Conversely, greater heart rate variability is associated with longevity. Decreased heart rate variability denotes the dominant influence of the sympathetic nervous system. Increased heart rate variability denotes the dominant influence of the parasympathetic nervous system. Sympathetic dominance (fight/flight response) causes increased muscle tension and decreased digestion and sleep. Muscular strength is needed to fight or run from the lion or bear, but not needed to digest or sleep during this time. Digestion and sleep (healing and repair) are controlled by the parasympathetic nervous system. A person has to have the flexibility in the nervous systems to switch from the sympathetic system when under an emergency to the parasympathetic for digestion and rest. What is happening today is that 4 out of 5 persons are locked into this sympathetic dominance and have lost the ability to maintain parasympathetic dominance that should be present the majority of the time. Sympathetic dominance results in tight, sore muscles, poor digestion, and poor sleep.

Sympathetic dominance produces adrenaline and cortisol, adrenaline and cortisol, and more adrenaline and cortisol. While this is good for the short term, it is devastating to body functions over an extended period of time. Chronic cortisol production produces insulin and thyroid receptor resistance, which are both epidemic in U.S. society today. Long term sympathetic dominance and elevated cortisol levels cause disease with psychological symptoms. The physiology of this sympathetic dominance places an individual in a catabolic state wherein tissue breaks down faster than it can be rebuilt. The modern physical environment of polluted air, water, food, and media creates an autonomic imbalance with sympathetic dominance. The good news is that you can take charge of your and your family's health.

First, I identify some of the problems and then present the solutions. Here are some of the conditions that very few people had 100 years ago or even prior to WWII but are rapidly increasing and common today. Since WWII, some 70,000+ chemicals have been introduced into the environment. Prior to that, there was less diabetes, obesity, cancer, autoimmune disease, allergies, and ADHD. The prevalence rates of these diseases pre-WWII were quite different than they are today.

Diabetes

Less than 1 % of the population had type II diabetes prior to WWII. Today approximately 12-14 % of the American population has type II diabetes.[1] Interestingly, there is a parallel graphing of the increased amount of chemical production, including herbicides and pesticides, and increased incidence of diabetes type II dating back to the 1940s.[2] Not only is type II diabetes increasing but the age of onset has become younger and younger. Once thought to be a disease associated with old age, it is now occurring in young adults and teenagers. Interestingly, the youngest patient recently documented with type II diabetes was a three and one-half year old in Texas.[3] The increased prevalence of type I diabetes positively correlates with the same timeline as well.[4] The prevalence of diabetes from 1940 has climbed from less than 5 per 100,000 to about 30 in 100,000 by 2010, a 600% increase.[2] The most recent U.S. data shows that the number of children with type 1 diabetes increased by 21% just between 2001 and 2009.[5]

The rise in the U.S is dwarfed by the rise in China, traditionally a country with low incidence. However, the incidence of type 1 diabetes in Shanghai's children increased by 14.2% per year between 1997 and 2011.[6] Between 2005 and 2020, the number of European children under 5 who will have type 1 diabetes is expected to double.[7] Additionally, there are the economic costs to consider. "It is estimated that type 1 diabetes costs the U.S. $14.4 billion in medical costs and lost income each year."[8] "In 2002, U.S. spending on diabetes (type 1 and type 2) was estimated to be $132 billion. Rising health care expenditures are a serious problem, and people with diabetes incur a significant portion of health care spending."[9]

Reference List

1. Menke A, Casagrande S, Cowie, CC. Prevalence of diabetes in adolescents aged 12 to 19 years in the United States, 2005-2014. *JAMA.* 2016 Jul 19;316(3):344-5. doi: 10.1001/jama.2016.8544.
2. Neel BA, Sargis RM. The paradox of progress: environmental disruption of metabolism and the diabetes epidemic. 2011. American Diabetes Association. http://diabetes.diabetesjournals.org/content/60/7/1838.long.
3. Susman E. Texas toddler diagnosed with type 2 diabetes. *MedpageToday.* https://www.medpagetoday.com/meetingcoverage/easd/53606. 2017. Accessed Nov 30, 2017.
4. Schmidt, MS. Questions persist: environmental factors in autoimmune disease. *Environ Health Perspect* 2011 June, 119 (6): A248-A253. doi: 10 1289/chp 119-a248.
5. Dabelea D, Mayer-Davis EJ, Saydah S, et. al. Prevalence of type 1 and type 2 diabetes among children and adolescents from 2001 to 2009. *JAMA.* 2014 May 7;311(17):1778-86. doi: 10.1001/jama.2014.3201.
6. Zhao H, Theinpont B, Yesilyurt BT, et. al. Mismatch repair deficiency endows tumors with a unique mutation signature and sensitivity to DNA double-strand breaks. *Elife.* 2014 Aug 1;3:e02725. doi: 10.7554/eLife.02725.
7. Patterson CC, Dahlquist GG, Gyürus E, et.al. Incidence trends childhood type 1 diabetes in Europe during 1989-2003 and predicted new cases 2005-20: a multicentre perspective registration study. *Lancet.* 2009 Jun 13;373(9680):2027-33. doi: 10.1016/S0140-6736(09)60568-7.
8. Tao B, Pietropaolo M, Atkinson M, Schatz D, Taylor D. Estimating the cost of type 1 diabetes in U.S.: a propensity score matching method. *PLoS One.* 2010; 5(7): e11501.
9. Hogan P, Dall T, Nikolov P. Economic costs of diabetes in the U.S. in 2002. *Diabetes Care: Alexandria* Vol 26 Iss 3 (Mar 2003): 917-32.

Obesity

An exhaustive search of studies shows very little reliable statistical data on the percentage of obesity in the United States pre-WWII. However, from the millions of photographs of large groups of people from this era, and the percentage of people who were obese in these photographs by today's standards is markedly less. I did find some data on eighteen-year-old men, admitted to the Citadel, a military academy in Charleston, South Carolina, who were born in in the 1920s—1930s compared to the US population in the 1950s and 1980's. The average BMI of a 70-inch tall young man were compared between these two periods of time. The BMI from the group born in 1920-1939 that was admitted into the Citadel varied very little from the group born in the 1950s. The average of both groups was very close: The Citadel group born during 1920-1939 averaged a BMI of 22.3, and the US population averaged a BMI of 22.4. This statistic jumps to a BMI of 24.2 in the group of eighteen-year-olds born in the 1980s. This correlates to an average increase in weight from about 155 pounds, which is what I weighed when graduating high school in 1973, to about 167 pounds for those born in the 1980s.

Additional data from 1960-1962 demonstrates some problem with being overweight with 44.8 % of the participants being considered overweight/obese with more men than women in this classification.[1] At the time, overweight was defined as a BMI of 25 or more, and obese was classified with a BMI of 30 or more.[2] In data from the years 1999-2000, the percentage of overweight/obesity increased to 64.5 % with a shift to more women than men. This is almost a 50% increase in the span of 40 years. More alarming is the increased incidence of obesity during this time from 13.3 % in 1960-1962 to 30.9 % in 1999-2000, an increase of 233 %.[1] While diet and exercise are important factors in the obesity epidemic, new research demonstrates that one contribution comes from the exposure of chemical obesogons. Food and beverages, including water, often contains obesogens. Chemicals known to disrupt hormones affect the size and number of fat cells or hormones that regulate appetite and metabolism. "Treating obesity and obesity-related conditions costs billions of dollars a year. By one estimate, the U.S. spent $190 billion on obesity-related health care expenses in 2005, which is double previous estimates."[3]

Reference List

1. Pastor PN, Makuc DM, Rueben C, Xia H . Chartbook on trends in the health of Americans: *Health, United States, 2002.* Hyattsville, MD: National Center for Health Statistics. https://www.cdc.gov/nchs/data/hus/hus02.pdf
2. Komlos J, Brabec M. The trend of mean BMI values of US adults, birth cohorts 1882-1986 indicates that the obesity epidemic began earlier than hitherto thought. *Am J Hum Biol.* 2010 Sep-Oct;22(5):631-8. doi: 10.1002/ajhb.21055.
3. Cawley J, Meyerhoefer C. The medical care costs of obesity: an instrumental variables approach. *J Health Econ.* 2012; 31:219-30.

Cancer

Depending upon the type of cancer, cancer mortality rates have increased by 50% since 1940, despite all the technologies available to us today. In 1930, 1 in 3,000 people were diagnosed with cancer. The mortality rate for all cancers was 97.4 per 100,000 people. In 1940, the mortality rate was 120.3 per 100, 000. The cancer mortality rate peaked in 1990 at 203.2 per 100, 000 and has slightly declined since then. It is now at about the same level it was in 1980. However, the number of people diagnosed with cancer has dramatically increased during this time, especially among the young.[1]

Today, an estimated "1 in 2 men and 1 in 3 women will be diagnosed with cancer during their lifetimes."[2] Tobacco smoke, nutrition, physical activity, and exposure to environmental carcinogens are estimated to be responsible for 75-80% of cancer diagnosis and death in the US. Occupational and environmental exposures linked to known, specific carcinogens are responsible for about 34,000 or 6% of cancer deaths per year. What is not well understood is the potential interaction of environmental carcinogens with genetic and lifestyle factors as well as the interaction of genetic and lifestyle factors in the development of cancer. Furthermore, since chemicals going into the environment are not exhaustively tested for their carcinogenicity, the cancer burden caused by exposures to environmental carcinogens may be even larger.[3]

In 2010, medical costs associated with cancer were projected to reach $124.6 billion with the highest costs associated with breast cancer ($16.5 billion), followed by colorectal cancer ($14 billion), lymphoma ($12 billion), lung cancer ($12 billion), and prostate cancer ($12 billion).[4] Based on growth and aging of the U.S. population, medical expenditures are projected to reach at least $158 billion in 2010 dollars—an increase of 27 %, according to an analysis by the National Institutes of Health. Researchers from the National Cancer Institute (NCI), a division of the NIH, claim that if newly developed tools for cancer diagnosis, treatment, and follow-up continue to be more expensive, medical expenditures for cancer could reach as high as $207 billion.[3]

Reference List

1. *Vital Statistics of the United States*; 1971-2001, U.S. National Center for Health Statistics, https://www.cdc.gov/nchs/products/vsus.htm & *National Vital Statistics Report (NVSR)* (formerly *Monthly Vital Statistics Report*). https://www.cdc.gov/nchs/nvss/index.htm. Accessed Dec 3, 2017.
2. Chusteka Z. Cancer strikes 1 in 2 men and 1 in 3 women. *News & Perspective.* Feb 9, 2007. https://www.medscape.com/viewarticle/551998. Accessed Jan 8, 2018.
3. Physicians for Social Responsibility. *Cancer and toxic chemicals.* Oct 9, 2013. http://www.psr.org/environment-and-health/confronting-toxics/cancer-and-toxic-chemicals.html. Accessed Jan 8, 2018.
4. National Institutes of Health. Cancer costs projected to reach at least $158 billion in 2020. *News Releases* Jan 12, 2011. https://www.nih.gov/news-events/news-releases/cancer-costs-projected-reach-least-158-billion-2020. Accessed Jan 9, 2018.

Allergies

Allergies and asthma have increased by approximately 300% since the mid-1990s. Food allergies are a growing public health concern: As many as fifteen million people have been diagnosed with IgE-type food allergies.[2] Symptoms of IgE reactions include coughing, sneezing, itchy and watery eyes, hives, and anaphylactic shock. "Today, an estimated nine million or 4% of adults in the U.A. have these kinds of allergies. Nearly six million or 8% of children in the U.S. also have these types of allergies with young children affected the most. Boys appear to develop food allergies more than girls."[2]

Other allergic conditions, such as atopic dermatitis and *eosinophilic* gastrointestinal diseases, may result from food allergies. Although childhood allergies to milk, egg, wheat, and soy generally resolve in childhood, they appear to be resolving more slowly than in previous decades with many children still allergic beyond age five. Allergies to peanuts, tree nuts, fish, or shellfish are generally lifelong allergies.[2] The above statistics only reflect a specific type of allergic reaction, which only reflects only a small percentage of the totality of all allergic and sensitivity reactions. There are multiple other types of allergic reactions, including IgA, IgM, and IgG type reactions. There are also sensitivity reactions that do not produce a true immune response but cause an inflammatory reaction of some kind in the body. Unfortunately, there is no reliable statistical data on the true prevalence of allergy/sensitivity in the U.S. and the world because of the lack of any form of unified testing. My clinical experience of 37 plus years and over 15,000 patients indicates that this lack of unified testing may be a problem in the majority of individuals to varying degrees as I have never tested a patient with IgG or MRT that did not have at least two or more allergies and/or sensitivities. Most of the time there were double-digit allergies/sensitivities in the patients I evaluated. Of course, all these patients exhibited signs and symptoms of chronic inflammation of some kind.

In today's world, I find there are more people by middle age than not who are taking some kind of stress medication that is causing inflammation, and here are the statistics. During 2011-2014 in a thirty-day period, 48.9% had used at least one prescription drug; 23.1% had used three or more prescription drugs; and 11.9% had used five or more prescription drugs.[4] Oftentimes, the source of the reoccurring stress causing inflammation, a condition that often prompts physicians to prescribe an antibiotic, is from a food/chemical allergy/sensitivity. The annual cost of allergies just related to children is $15 billion each year in Canada.[5] In 2007, the last year that data was available, the total incremental cost of asthma alone to society was $56 billion.[6]

Reference List

1. Branum A, Lukacs S. Food allergy among U.S. children: trends in prevalence and hospitalizations. *National Center for Health Statistics Data Brief.* http://www.cdc.gov/nchs/data/databriefs/db10.htm. Accessed Dec 4, 2017.
2. Food Allergy Research and Education. *Food allergy facts and statistics for the U.S.* https://www.foodallergy.org/sites/default/files/migrated-files/file/facts-stats.pdf. Accessed Dec 11, 2017.
3. Kattan JD, Cocco RR, Järvinen KM. Milk and soy allergy. *Pediatr Clin North Am.* 2011 Apr; 58(2): 407–426. doi: 10.1016/j.pcl.2011.02.005.
4. Center for Disease Control and Prevention. Therapeutic drug use. *National Center for Health Statistics.* May 3, 2017. https://www.cdc.gov/nchs/fastats/drug-use-therapeutic.htm. Accessed Jan 9, 2018.
5. CHILD Study. *Canadian Healthy Infant Longitudinal Development Study.* 2013. http://www.canadianchildstudy.ca/project_deliverables.html. Accessed Jan 9, 2018.
6. Nunes C, Pereira AM, Morais-Almeida M. Asthma cost and social impact. *Asthma Res Pract.* 2017; 3: 1. https://www.ncbi.nlm.nih.gov/pmc/articles/PMC5219738/. Accessed Jan 9, 2018.

ADHD

Both of my parents were schoolteachers, and my maternal grandmother began teaching grades 1-8 at the age of 15 in 1913. Because of this, I was very aware at an early age of acceptable classroom behaviour. Sometimes one child in a class of twenty-five was termed "hyper" in grade school as I recall. Although the classification has changed in the years, there was definitely a decrease in the number of children with learning and behavioural challenges pre-WWII. My first partner in practice who also was a classmate had five children, one of which had some behaviour problems that could be classified as ADHD today and which were improved by following the Feingold diet (avoiding processed foods with food dyes and the like). This was in the late 70s and early 80s. In 1980, the term was ADD (Attention Deficit Disorder). Although the disorder is now recognized as having different forms, there is evidence of this condition having occurred in children dating back to before 1900. The prevalence has steadily increased, particularly in the last eight years, by a startling 42 % increase. "Before 1900, symptoms of ADHD were considered a moral problem of children or their parents, and discipline or punishment was seen as the best treatment. In 1902, Sir George Still described ADHD as a behavioural disorder that may be inherited. Around 1919, some survivors of the influenza pandemic developed encephalitis and showed symptoms of ADHD, so the condition was then blamed on brain damage.

"In 1940, symptoms of ADHD continued to be blamed on 'minimal brain damage.' In 1968, a disorder similar to ADHD, called 'hyperkinetic reaction of childhood,' appeared in the *Diagnostic and Statistical Manual of Mental Disorders* for the first time. In 1979, an article in the influential, *Science,* referred to "the hyperactive child syndrome." In 1980, the third edition of the manual used the name 'attention deficit disorder' (ADD). By 1994, the manual's fourth edition recognized the disorder as 'attention deficit hyperactivity disorder,' with three subgroups."[1] Today, 'males are almost three times more likely to be diagnosed with ADHD than females":[2] This means that 12.9% of men will be diagnosed with the attention disorder, and 4.9 % of women will be diagnosed during their lifetimes. While symptoms of ADHD typically first appear between the ages of 3 and 6, the average age of ADHD diagnosis is at seven years old. However, the diagnosis of ADHD has now been extended to adults with about 4% of U.S. adults over the age of 18 diagnosed with ADHD. The American Psychiatric Association (APA) estimates that 5% of American children have ADHD while the Center for Disease Control and Prevention (CDC) estimates the number at more than double that with 11% of American children ages 4 to 17 with the disorder. If this is correct, that represents an increase of 42% in just 8 years.[2]

Reference List

1. Iliades C. The past, present, and future of ADHD. *Everyday Health.* Aug 31, 2010. https://www.everydayhealth.com/adhd-awareness/an-adhd-timeline.aspx. Accessed Jan 9, 2018.
2. Holland K, Riley E. *ADHD by the numbers: facts, statistics, and you.* https://www.healthline.com/health/adhd/facts-statistics-infographic. Published Sep 4, 2014. Accessed Dec 6, 2017.

Autoimmune Diseases

During my practice in the 1980s, I recall only the occasional patient with rheumatoid arthritis or celiac disease. Today, I see more patients diagnosed with autoimmune diseases (AD) than any other conditions. These conditions were uncommon in the U.S. prior to WWII. In the past 40 years, the estimate for the increase of autoimmune and autoimmune-like diseases ranges from 90% to 600%. According to Mayo Clinic researchers, the incidence of lupus has nearly tripled in the U. S, during this same time period.[1] Additional international studies indicate that autoimmune diseases, such as lupus, multiple sclerosis (MS), scleroderma, to name a few, have also increased since the 1970s. The American Autoimmune Related Diseases Association recognizes 100 autoimmune diseases.[2] The National Institute of Health (NIH) estimates the number of people in the U.S. with AD as 23 and ½ million while people with cancer stands at 9 million, and those with heart disease is 22 million.[3] The American Autoimmune Related Diseases Association (AARDA) calculates that 50 million people in the U.S suffer from autoimmune disease.[2]

The difference between the two statistics can be explained by how each group defines AD and how they collect their data. The NIH numbers only include 24 diseases for which good epidemiology studies were available. Taken collectively, these diseases that also include Type 1 diabetes, Hashimoto's disease, Graves' disease, vasculitis, myasthenia gravis, connective tissue diseases, autoimmune Addison's disease, vitiligo, rheumatoid arthritis, hemolytic anemia, celiac disease, and scleroderma are now the second highest cause of chronic illness in the U.S. and the third leading cause of Social Security disability, behind heart disease and cancer. Acquired Immune Deficiency Syndrome (AIDS) is not an autoimmune disease because a virus attacks the autoimmune system. In contrast, with autoimmune diseases the tissues of the body become the casualty of friendly fire for what was intended for a foreign invader.

Autoimmune diseases are the eighth leading cause of death among women,[4] shortening the average woman's lifespan by 15 years.[5] Not surprisingly, the economic burden to the U.S. is staggering. Autoimmune diseases represent a yearly health-care burden of more than $120 billion, compared to the yearly health-care burden of $70 billion for direct medical costs for cancer. To re-emphasize the numbers, consider that while 2.2 million women are living with breast cancer and 7.2 million women have coronary disease, an estimated 9.8 million women are afflicted with one of the seven more common autoimmune diseases: lupus, scleroderma, rheumatoid arthritis, multiple sclerosis, inflammatory bowel disease, Sjogren's Syndrome, and Type 1 Diabetes.[1] And all of these can lead to potentially fatal complications.

Having been in practice since 1980, I have observed the drastic increase in incidence of all the diseases above in the population. Not only is the incidence increasing for chronic illness and disease at an alarming rate, but also the age of onset is becoming younger and younger. Illnesses and diseases long associated with old age when I began practice are now occurring in young adults and even children.

One of the first things I do for many of my patients who are suffering from chronic inflammation, which is associated with all chronic illness/disease, is to assess one of the nine variables in health, diet— what they are eating. I want to know what food/chemical allergy/sensitivity they have. You will notice I did not say I want to find out *if* they have food/chemical allergy/sensitivity because everyone who is chronically ill does. It is a matter of how many and the severity. I have never tested a patient yet who did not have some food/chemical allergy/sensitivity.

Because of a failure to test or the different testing methods used by different practitioners, it is difficult to evaluate an accurate incidence of all the types of reactions. However, one of the more common tests performed by allergists is the RAST test, which consist of a scratch test on the skin. This type of test only checks for IgE-type reactions that are the type that causes coughing, sneezing, watery eyes, hives, or anaphylactic shock. As mentioned previously, there are many other types of allergies: IgA, IgM, and IgG, to name a few. Existing evidence suggests that the RAST test is a poor method for evaluating food allergies. Despite this blatant lack of appropriate testing, the statistics of documented food allergies are alarming, and this probably only represents a small percentage of true levels.

Reference List

1.   Nagazawa DJ. *The autoimmune epidemic: bodies gone haywire in a world out of balance—and the cutting edge science that promises hope.* New York: Touchstone; 2008.
2.   The American Autoimmune Related Diseases Association. *Autoimmune disease list.* https://www.aarda.org/diseaselist/. Published 2018. Accessed Jan 9, 2018.
3.   National Institute of Health. *Estimates of funding for various research, condition, and disease categories.* July 3, 2017. https://report.nih.gov/categorical_spending.aspx. Accessed Jan 9, 2018.
4.   Nelson R. Autoimmune diseases among top killers of younger women. *WebMD.* Sep 1, 2000. https://www.webmd.com/women/news/20000901/autoimmune-diseases-among-top-killers-of-younger-women#1. Accessed Jan 9, 2018.
5.   Rheumatoid Arthritis Support Network. *Rheumatoid arthritis life expectancy.* Aug 3, 2016. https://www.rheumatoidarthritis.org/ra/prognosis/life-expectancy/. Published Aug 3, 2016. Accessed Jan 9, 2018.
6.   Taylor SL. Food allergy—enigma and some potential solutions. *Journal of Food Protection* Apr 1980 43 (4): 300-306. http://jfoodprotection.org/doi/pdf/10.4315/0362-028X-43.4.300?code=fopr-site.

Chapter 2: Food/Chemical Allergy/Sensitivity

Here is a simple rule for eating. If the food you are eating was not available for your great-grandmother/father or great-great grandmother/father to eat (depending on your current age), you need to think twice about eating it. There are multiple differences in what they ate and what we eat. According to the World Health Organization (WHO), the vitamin/mineral content of the soil was about seven times greater 100 years ago than it is now. The average orange contained about 50 mg of Vitamin C just some 60 years ago. Today, the average orange contains about 5 mg of Vitamin C.[1] A hundred years ago, people in the U.S. did not have the belief that fat in real food was bad for you. They did not have hydrogenated oils and trans-fats. They did not have MSG. They did not have high fructose corn syrup. They did not have Ho-Ho's, Ding-Dongs, corn chips, pre-packaged potato chips, quart sized sodas, artificial sweeteners, and on and on. The amount of pesticides and herbicides in the food was negligible. All this has occurred since WWII.

A hundred years ago, people did not have GMO foods. Since the introduction of GMO foods in the 1990s, the use of Roundup, an herbicide, has increased 400% due to the weeds becoming increasingly resistant to this herbicide. I discuss this topic later in the book. I have devoted an entire chapter to glyphosates (Roundup), perhaps the single worse environmental stressor today. All of these combined changes have increased the likelihood of food and chemical allergy or sensitivity.

Mediator Release Testing (MRT) To the Rescue

MRT is my favorite go-to test to assess food and chemical allergies and sensitivities because it has 94% reliability for accuracy. Since there are many different types of immune and inflammatory responses in the body, it is absolutely imperative to know if you have a life-threatening IgE-type reaction, such as might occur with a peanut allergy that can quickly close off breathing passages. However, the vast majority of negative responses to these allergies and sensitivities occur anywhere from 2 or 3 hours to 72 hours later. Because of this time delay, it is more difficult to associate the symptoms with the offending food and/or chemical. The advantage of MRT is that is measures all reactions that cause inflammation, and, more importantly, it quantitates them.

By the time that I had reached my mid-fifties I had an increasing problem with rapid weight gain of five to eight pounds in a 24-48-hour period. An inflammatory reaction was the only possible cause. When I ordered the MRT on myself, I found the answers. I was most sensitive to sulfites, which were in most wines that I drank on weekends. I had also been trying to eat gluten-free and was having pancakes made from tapioca flour on the weekends. I was sensitive to tapioca. There were a couple of other foods and chemicals I was ingesting fairly regularly as well, such as oranges and tomatoes that I was reactive to. Once I stopped ingesting the reactive foods and chemicals I lost ten pounds in two to three weeks without cutting any calories.

MRT should be part of an evaluation for any patient who has any kind of chronic or reoccurring inflammation symptoms in their body. This inflammation could be in the form of gastritis, colitis, esophagitis, dermatitis, arthritis, cystitis, iritis, or any other kind of -itis you could think of or name. It should be a consideration for all children and adults who suffer from psychological symptoms, ADHD, and Autism Spectrum Disorder. For more information read my forthcoming book, *Raising a Healthy Baby & Child in Today's World.* MRT should be a consideration for weight loss/management. For more information read my forthcoming book, *Why Can't I Lose Weight?* MRT should be a consideration for any competitive athlete who wants to optimize his/her performance. For more information read my forthcoming book, *22 Tests Your Physician Never Heard of That Can Change/Save Your Life.* MRT should be part of a consideration for any individual who wants to reduce stress and optimize functional longevity in their lives.

Another reason I choose MRT to confirm these allergies and sensitivities with patients is that it has extremely high-reliability and reproducibility. It also has a quick turn-around time of 7-10 days, is easy-to-read, and provides extensive detailed reports that provide sufficient information to educate the patient about different food choices. The report quantifies the relative inflammatory reactivity of each food and chemical the patient has. Not only are moderate and severe foods/chemical identified, but also the patient also has a list of ideal foods to minimize inflammation. MRT explains the ideal foods for the patient to eat to produce less stress and inflammation.

Instead of what the patient can't eat, I tell my patients to pick foods they are the least reactive to on the list and eat just those for 30 days. Then I recommend something like Liposome Colostrum or a combination of l-glutamine, arabinogalactans, aloe vera leaf extract, slipper elm, and marshmallow to help heal the leaky gut.

Many physicians use elimination diets to try to figure out what causes the negative symptoms. This can work if there are only a small number of offending foods. However, it has been my experience that most people tested have double-digit food allergies and sensitivities, making an elimination diet almost impossible for figuring out which foods are causing the problem. Many other physicians order IgE, IgA, IgM, or IgG testing as I have in the past. Each of these evaluates a different specific type of allergic reaction. IgE reactions are the smallest percentage of all of these. However, they can be quite severe and occur quickly, causing anaphylactic shock and even death. People with these types of allergies usually carry an epi (short for epinephrine or adrenaline) pin with them for such emergencies.

The other type of allergic reactions besides the IgE type take longer to manifest, sometimes up to 72 hours in the case of an IgG reaction. With a longer timeframe before the reaction occurs, it is much more difficult for an individual to associate his/her symptoms with a food or foods they ate up to 3 days prior. Also, an individual may not even associate the headache, lethargy, sleepiness, or loose stool they are experiencing with any food or chemical ingested 24-72 hours earlier. Not only does MRT identify any allergic reaction, but it also picks up any other type of inflammatory reaction. MRT prevents loss of time and productivity and reduces the frustration of the elimination diet by quickly identifying offending foods and chemicals.

Inflammation has been reliably identified as the cause or, at the very least, a significant contributory factor to all chronic illness. Human bodies fight inflammation with hormones like DHEA, testosterone, estradiol, and cortisol (read *13 Secrets to Optimal Aging*), and antioxidant micronutrients (read *Micronutrient Testing*). When there is excess chronic inflammation, hormone and micronutrient levels become depleted over time, causing a chronic –

itis of some kind and ultimately degenerative disease. It is critical to reduce or minimize the excess or reoccurring inflammation to avoid depletion of hormone and micronutrient levels. Reducing inflammation-causing reactive foods is essential to reducing stress on the body and for promoting optimum health and longevity.

Food sensitivities often play a role in many common health conditions. Chronic health complaints, such as digestive problems, headaches, joint and muscle pain, and fatigue, are all symptoms that can be caused by the immune system's reaction to foods, additives, or other dietary substances. Sometimes the reactive food is something easy to identify like milk. Other times it's a food chemical like solanine, which is anything but easy to determine. The problem is that any food or food additive can be reactive. Even foods that are considered "healthy," such as chicken, broccoli, or garlic can cause symptoms. Often, there are many reactive foods or chemicals, not just one or two. In addition, reactions can be delayed and/or dose-dependent. This means you may not feel the effects of a reaction until many hours or days after you've eaten the reactive foods, or unless you eat enough of the reactive food. For all of these reasons, dealing with food sensitivities on your own is very difficult.

If you have some kind of chronic inflammation, the first thing you need to do is identify which foods and food chemicals are causing you problems. MRT, the most accurate test available to identify foods, additives and chemicals causing sensitivity reactions, can do this.

The following information is used with the permission of Oxford Biomedical Technologies. Additional information can be obtained at this website: http://nowleap.com/the-patented-mediator-release-test-mrt/.

MRT Reaction Categories

MRT quantifies the level of reactivity and breaks reactions into 3 categories: Non-Reactive (GREEN), Moderately Reactive (YELLOW), and Reactive (RED).

- **Green**: The substances in this category show the lowest degree of reactivity. Foods from this category (with the exception of known allergic or intolerant foods) will comprise the first phases of your eating plan.
- **Yellow**: These substances show relatively less reactivity than the RED category but should also be strictly avoided. Clinical experience has shown that substances within this category may provoke symptoms alone, when eaten in combination, or when over-consumed.
- **Red**: These substances show the highest relative level of reactivity and are the most likely to be contributing directly to your health problems. It is important to avoid these foods and chemicals strictly. The LEAP lmmunoCalm Dietary Program was developed by a team of dieticians, physicians, immunologists, and other health professionals drawing on over 100 years combined experience treating the health problems associated with food sensitivities. They encourage you to get the most out of your efforts by following these guidelines strictly and working closely with your healthcare provider, who may customize your plan to meet your special needs. The closer you follow your plan the more health benefits you receive.

Understanding Your MRT Results

MRT is a patented blood test (U.S. Patent numbers 6,1114, 174 & 6,200,815) that quantifies how strongly your immune cells react to the foods and food chemicals tested by measuring *intracellular mediator release* indirectly. When released from immune cells, chemical *mediators* such as *histamine, cytokines,* and *prostaglandins* produce damaging effects on body tissues that lead to the development of symptoms. Identifying harmful substances is the first step towards improving your health if you suffer from food sensitivities. The next step involves following an individualized eating plan that systematically builds a healthy diet of foods that you can actually tolerate. It has been my experience that most patients experience positive results within 2 weeks after removing reactive foods from their diets.

A distinctive feature of food sensitivities is that almost any food or chemical can potentially be reactive and a specific food may cause a problem with one person but not another. The individualized nature of sensitivity reactions means an individualized approach is most appropriate and most effective. The results of your MRT testing combined with other dietary information provided by you are used to develop a food reintroduction schedule specifically for you. Each phase of the reintroduction schedule corresponds to a time frame that specifies when and how to reintroduce the listed foods into your diet.

In summary, when a person has food sensitivities, the first step in getting better is to identify reactive foods and chemicals. The next step is to figure out what to eat and how to eat. It has been my experience that most patients experience positive results within two weeks of removing reactive foods from their diets.

Chapter 3: Heavy Metals

Heavy metal poisoning from cadmium, lead, arsenic, aluminum, and others, especially mercury, may be more prevalent than anyone suspected. To my knowledge, there have not been multiple studies on a general population to determine if heavy metal toxicities exist in a large percentage of the population. However, in 2007, 1,000 people gathered for a four-day health seminar related to mercury testing. Of the 1,000 attendees, 680 men and women from the ages of 18 to 70 who lived throughout the U. S. and Canada were tested. An alarming 95% of the people tested with body mercury levels in the 'Elevated' or 'Very Elevated' reference range, and just 5% tested in the 'Green', or 0 reference range.[1]

Cadmium and lead can be found in automobile and industrial vapors, and lead may come from dental fillings with lead contamination from lead-based paints. Aluminum toxicity can occur secondary to exposure to aluminum cookware and cans. Arsenic is frequently found in well water. Of all these, mercury seems to be most prevalent. In 1991, the WHO confirmed that mercury contained in dental amalgam is the greatest source of mercury vapor in non-industrialized settings exposing the concerned population to mercury levels significantly exceeding those set for food and for air. But these "silver" fillings are not the only source of mercury. Certain types and brands of the following common products also may contain mercury: fish, thermometers, button cell batteries, skin crèmes, vaccines, barometers, cosmetics, tattoos, thermostats, light-up sports shoes, disinfectants, fluorescent light bulbs, and high fructose corn syrup.

Exposure to mercury can occur in a number of ways. One may come into contact with mercury or its fumes from broken thermometers and other spills in the home, school, or workplace or breathe in airborne mercury from a coal burning power plant, mining operations, or industrial sources. Thousands of people work in an occupation that uses mercury, such as a dental office or manufacturing plant. Millions are exposed daily by eating fish that have been contaminated with methyl mercury. In general, the larger the fish, the more susceptible it is to mercury contamination. Different regions around the world have different fish on the "consumer beware" list, but a few of the most at risk are shark, swordfish, grouper, tuna, Chilean sea bass, marlin, tilefish, and farmed salmon.

However, in today's world, one of the greatest risks for ongoing mercury toxicity occurs from vaccines, especially for the young. The numbers and recommended schedules of vaccinations continue to increase. Mercury, added to extend the shelf life, adds not value to the vaccine itself. Instead, it is a neurotoxin that can cause permanent neurological and immune damage and fetal death. Every time you receive tetanus or flu shot you receive more mercury. There is no doubt in my mind that this practice has caused the loss of quality of life for hundreds or thousands of people. Due to pressure from the public, some companies have reported not using mercury in the vaccines because they have substituted aluminum. Many people believe that Thermosil, which contains methyl mercury, was eliminated in childhood vaccinations in 1999. What happened is that the FDA allowed a label change so that manufacturers no longer have to list Thermosil as an ingredient unless it is used as a preservative. According to the FDA, if Thermosil is used only in the manufacturing process, the vaccine may be labeled "Thermosil-free."

In reality, some vaccines, including the DTaP (diphtheria, tetanus, and pertussis) vaccine, DT (diphtheria) vaccine, the Haemophilus influenzae type b vaccines of Hib, ACTHib, TriHIBit, and Meningococcal vaccine,[2] still given to infants and children contain this toxin. Vaccines for tetanus, influenza, and meningococcal containing ethyl mercury are still given to children, pregnant women, and other adults.[2] Vaccines using aluminum adjuvants include those for hepatitis A, hepatitis B, diphtheria-tetanus, Haemophilus influenza type b, and pneumococcal. However, the live viral vaccines for measles, mumps, rubella, varicella, and rotavirus do not us this additive.

Recent lab tests conducted at the *Natural News* Forensic Food lab revealed that seasonal flu vaccines that are pushed on virtually everyone these days, including young babies, pregnant women, and the elderly,[3] contain excessive high levels of neurotoxic mercury. The lab tests of vials of batch flu vaccine produced by British pharmaceutical giant GlaxoSmithKline (GSK) found them to contain upwards of 51 parts per million of mercury or 25,000 times the legal maximum for drinking water as established by the Environmental Protection Agency (EPA).[4]

Some vaccines contain both mercury and aluminum as preservatives, increasing neurological damage risk exponentially. Not only can aluminum damage the brain of an infant or child, but it also accumulates in the brain: It has been found in the brains of Alzheimer's patients, for example. Mercury or arsenic toxicity can interfere with thyroid function, and thyroid hypofunction is epidemic in the adult population in the US. Thyroid function is critical to the function of every cell and for signaling the adrenal glands and the gonads (testicles/ovaries). There are over 300 different symptoms related to low thyroid function that can occur from heavy metal poisoning (as well as other conditions). Mercury toxicity definitely is a potential stress in many people. The majority of the patients I have tested, including myself, have toxic levels of mercury in their bodies.

Symptoms of Chronic Mercury Poisoning

Body Function	Symptoms

Central nervous system	Irritability
	Anxiety/nervousness, often with difficulty in breathing
	Restlessness
	Exaggerated response to stimulation
	Fearfulness
	Emotional instability
	    -lack of self-control
	    -fits of anger, with violent, irrational behavior
	Loss of self confidence
	Indecision
	Shyness or timidity, being easily embarrassed
	Loss of memory
	Inability to concentrate
	Lethargy/drowsiness
	Insomnia
	Mental depression, despondency
	Withdrawal

	Suicidal tendencies
	Manic depression
	Numbness and tingling of hands, feet, fingers, toes, or lips
	Muscle weakness progressing to paralysis
	Ataxia
	Tremors/trembling of hands, feet, lips, eyelids or tongue
	Incoordination
	Monaural transmission failure resembling Myasthenia Gravis
	Motor neuron disease (ALS)
	Multiple Sclerosis
Head, neck, oral cavity disorders	Bleeding gums
	Alveolar bone loss
	Loosening of teeth
	Excessive salivation
	Foul breath
	Metallic taste
	Burning sensation, with tingling of lips, face
	Tissue pigmentation (amalgam tattoo of gums)
	Leukoplakia
	Stomatitis (sores in the mouth)
	Ulceration of gingiva, palate, tongue
	Dizziness/acute, chronic vertigo
	Ringing in the ears
	Hearing difficulties
Gastrointestinal	Food sensitivities, especially to milk and eggs
	Abdominal cramps, colitis, diverticulitis or other G.I. complaint
	Chronic diarrhea/constipation
Cardiovascular	Abnormal heart rhythm
	Characteristic findings on EKG
	-abnormal changes in the S-T

	segment and/or -lower broadened P wave Unexplained elevated serum triglyceride Unexplained elevated cholesterol Abnormal blood pressure, either high or low

Immunologic	Repeated infections
	   -viral and fungal
	   -mycobacteria
	   -candida and other yeast infections
	Cancer
	Autoimmune disorders
	   -arthritis
	   -lupus erythematous (LE)
	   -multiple sclerosis (MS)
	   -scleroderma
	   -amyolateral sclerosis (ALS)
	   -hypothyroidism

Systemic	Chronic headaches
	Allergies
	Severe dermatitis
	Unexplained reactivity
	Thyroid disturbance
	Subnormal body temperature
	Cold, clammy skin, especially hands and feet
	Excessive perspiration, w/frequent night sweats
	Unexplained sensory symptoms, including pain
	Unexplained numbness or burning sensations
	Unexplained anemia
	G-6-PD deficiency
	Chronic kidney disease
	   -nephrotic syndrome
	   -receiving renal dialysis

	-kidney infection -adrenal disease General fatigue Loss of appetite/with or without weight loss Loss of weight Hypoglycemia

Reference List

1. Healing the eye and wellness center. *The MercOut detoxification program: the safe effective way to free your body of mercury.* 2017. http://www.healingtheeye.com/mercout.html. Accessed 8 December 2017.
2. Piper-Terry M. *Tag archives: Marcella Piper-Terry: did you know? a few facts about vaccines.* Aug 8, 2012. http://vaxtruth.org/tag/marcella-piper-terry/. Accessed 8 Dec 2017.
3. Centers for Disease Control and Prevention. *Key facts about influenza (flu).* Oct 3, 2017. https://www.cdc.gov/flu/keyfacts.htm. Accessed Jan 12, 2018.
4. Adams M. *Exclusive: natural news tests flu vaccine for heavy metals, finds 25,000 times higher mercury level than EPA limit for water.* June 3, 2014. https://www.naturalnews.com/045418_flu_shots_influenza_vacc ines_mercury.html. Accessed 11 Dec 2017.
5. Queen HL. *Chronic mercury toxicity: new hope against an endemic disease (doctor's guide to lifestyle counseling).* Colorado Springs, CO: Queen and Company Health Communications; 1988.
6. MercuryTalk.com. *Testing for mercury toxicity.* http://mercurytalk.com/articles/Testing-for-Mercury-Toxicity.html#.WispolVrxPs.2015. Accessed 8 December 2017.

Aluminum Toxicity

Aluminum is the third most abundant element on the planet and represents about 8% of total minerals. Because it is very reactive, it is always found in combination with other minerals. It occurs naturally in water and animal and plant tissues.[1] While aluminum is environmentally abundant, it is not necessary for life. In fact, it "is a widely recognized neurotoxin that inhibits more than 200 biologically important functions and causes various adverse effects in plants, animals, and humans."[2] Since it is ubiquitous in most foods and drinks, including drinking water (sometimes used in treatment facilities), fruit juices, wine, and beer, you likely ingest aluminum compounds on a daily basis.

In addition to occurring naturally, it is a component in many manufactured materials, including cosmetics[3, 4] prescription pharmaceuticals and over-the-counter drugs,[4] such as local therapeutic agents, anti-diarrheal drugs, or antacids. The connection between aluminum and Alzheimer's disease was first discussed in the 1960s. While this has been controversial, new research shows aluminum connects with metal-binding proteins, particularly in the brain. Studies in Canada, England, Wales, Norway, and France found that aluminum contamination of drinking water was associated with dementia and cognitive decline.[2] The presence of high concentrations of aluminum has now been verified in brain tissue of 12 donors diagnosed with familial Alzheimer's disease.[5] These findings reflect those of an earlier case study of a sixty-six-year-old man who died of early onset aggressive form of Alzheimer's disease. This disease was the result of inhaling aluminum dust.[6] Inhaling aluminum dust or vapors sends these particles directly into the lungs in a highly absorbable form, where the particles pass into the bloodstream and are distributed throughout the body, including bones and brain.

The dangers of aluminum powder inhalation have been known for over 50 years. It is associated with pulmonary fibrosis and encephalopathy.[7] Aluminum factory workers have an increased incidence of asthma.[8] According to a Public Health Statement on aluminum based on recommendations of the Environmental Protection Agency, if you are exposed to aluminum, many factors, including the dose, duration, and how you came in contact with it, will determine whether you will be harmed. "You must also consider any other chemicals you are exposed to and your age, sex, diet, family traits, lifestyle, and state of health."[9] If you live in an industrial area, your exposure is higher than average.[9] In the Tampa Bay area where I practice, environmental aluminum levels that translate into patient levels are some of the highest in the country

---

and more concentrated than in the rest of the state, except for the Miami area.

According to the CDC, the average adult in the U.S. consumes about 7 to 9 mg of aluminum per day in food and in lesser amounts from air and water. Fortunately, only about 1% of the aluminum ingested orally actually is absorbed into the body.[9] A well-functioning digestive tract and kidneys remove the remainder. I want to stress the importance of properly functioning kidneys for this process.

When tested in a lab, aluminum contamination has been found in a vast number of products on the market from foods and beverages to pharmaceuticals. Not too surprisingly given it prevalence in the environment, aluminum has been found in all of the follow products. Some of these have been mentioned previously.

Foods, such as baking powder, self-rising flour, salt, baby formula, coffee creamers, baked and processed foods, and coloring and caking agents

Drugs, such as antacids, analgesics, and anti-diarrhea medications

Additives, such as magnesium stearate

Vaccines, such as Hepatitis A and B, Hib, DTap (diphtheria, tetanus, pertussis), pneumococcal vaccine, and Gardasit (HPV)

Cosmetics and personal care products, such as antiperspirants, deodorants (including salt crystals made of alum), lotions, sunscreens, and shampoos

Aluminum products, including foil, cans, juice pouches, tins, and water bottles [10, 12]

Tobacco and cannabis[11]

This level of contamination suggests that the manufacturing process itself is a significant part of the process. In one study, researchers analyzed 1,431 non-animal foods and beverages for aluminum content. They found that 77.8% of the analyzed items had an aluminum concentration between 0 to 10 mg/kg, 17.5% had aluminum concentrations between 10 to 100 mg/kg, and 4.6% had aluminum concentrations exceeding 100 mg/kg.[13]

To recap, aluminum compounds are often used as additive in foodstuffs and other household items. Additional contamination occurs when food comes into contact with aluminum equipment or foil because aluminum is unstable in the presence of acids and bases.

While aluminum equipment has a protective oxide film, this can be damaged from normal usage. Baked goods may contain high aluminum concentrations if baked and stored with aluminum utensils. Cooking food in aluminum foil significant increases contamination. Apparently, the more fat a meat contains the more aluminum is absorbed. According to a 2006 study, cooking meat in aluminum foil showed an increase in aluminum by 89% to 378%. Cooking poultry increased aluminum by 76% to 214%. Higher temperatures and cooking times contribute to the absorption of aluminum.[14] As with many toxins, it is the *cumulative effect* of many small exposures over time that leads to a toxic metal overload that undermines your health.

Although total elimination of aluminum is probably impossible, it can be markedly reduced by proper water filtration systems containing the NSF/ANSI 401 certification, air purification systems using the ActivePure[TM] NASA approved technology, and avoiding using aluminum cook ware and foil, deodorants and other personal products that contain aluminum, and unnecessary vaccines. Mercury and aluminum are two of the top offenders in the heavy metal toxicity category that cause neurological damage to fetuses, children, and adults. Continued use of vaccines as currently manufactured with mercury and/or aluminum should be strongly questioned. Wherever possible, eliminate products containing aluminum from your personal use. Repeated exposure has a cumulative negative effect.

Heavy metal toxicity is far too common. Every patient I have ever tested had some elevated levels of one or more heavy metals. As I stated previously, when I tested myself, I had elevated levels of mercury, lead, cadmium, and antimony. To reduce this heavy metal contamination, I immediately began taking specific supplements to chelate the heavy metals. Subsequent retesting has shown a marked reduction. If you have one of the following conditions, I strongly recommend you get heavy metal testing.

Toxic Element Exposure
Alopecia
Bone Density
Cardiovascular Disease
Depression
Dermatitis or Poor Wound Healing

Detoxification Therapy
Fatigue
Gastrointestinal Symptoms
Hypertension
Immune Function
Impaired Glucose Tolerance
Inflammation
Kidney Function
Nutritional Deficiencies
Parkinson's-like Symptoms

Reference List

1. Bernardo JF. Aluminum toxicity. *Medscape.* July 10, 2017. https://emedicine.medscape.com/article/165315-overview. P. Accessed Jan 12, 2018.
2. Kawahara M, Kato-Nigeshi M. Link between aluminum and the pathogenesis of Alzheimer's disease: the integration of aluminum and amyloid cascade hypotheses. *Int J Alzheimers Dis* 2011; 2011:276393. doi: 10.4061/2011/276393.
3. Rosenstein J. *7 controversial beauty ingredients you should know about.* Jan 3, 2016. https://www.allure.com/story/beauty-ingredients-to-avoid. Accessed Jan 12, 2018.
4. Aggrawal M, Rohrer J. Determination of aluminum in OTC pharmaceutical products. *Thermo Scientific.* https://assets.thermofisher.com/TFS-Assets/CMD/Application-Notes/AN-1142-IC-Aluminum-OTC-Pharmaceuticals-AN71750-EN.pdf. Accessed Jan 12, 2018.
5. Mirza A, King A, Troakes C, Exley C. *Aluminum in brain tissue in familial Alzheimer's disease.* 2016. https://www.sciencedirect.com/science/article/pii/S0946672X16 303777. Accessed Jan 12, 2018.
6. Exley C, Vickers T. Elevated brain aluminum and early onset Alzheimer's disease in an individual occupationally exposed to aluminum: a case report. *J Med Case Rep* 2014 Feb 10(8): 41. doi: 10.1186/1752-1947-8-41.
7. Mclaughlin AIG, Kazantzis G, King E, Teare D, Porter RJ, Owen R. Pulmonary fibrosis and encephalopathy associated with the inhalation of aluminum dust. *Brit J Industr Med* 1962

19: 253. http://oem.bmj.com/content/oemed/19/4/253.full.pdf. Accessed Jan 12, 2018.

8. Kongerud J, Soseth V. Respiratory disorders in aluminum smelter workers. *J Occup Environ Med* 2014 May; 56(5 Suppl): S60-S70. doi: 10.1097/JOM.0000000000000105.

9. Agency for Toxic Substances & Disease Registry. *Public health statement for aluminum.* Sep 2008. https://www.atsdr.cdc.gov/PHS/PHS.asp?id=1076&tid=34. Accessed Jan 12, 2018.

10. Analytical Research Labs. *Aluminum toxicity.* 2012. http://www.arltma.com/Articles/AlumToxDoc.htm. Accessed Jan 13, 2018.

11. Exley C, Begum A, Woolley MP, Bloor RN. Aluminum in tobacco and cannabis and smoking-related disease. *Am J Med* 2006 Mar, 119(3):276e9-11. doi: 10.1016/j.amjmed.2005.08.004.

12. Stahl T, Tashan H, Brunn H. Aluminum content of selected foods and food products. *Environ Sci Eur* Dec 2011 23:27.

13. Health and Natural Medicine. *New study the farmacy: Alzheimer's & aluminum link can no longer be ignored.* June 20, 2016. http://healthandnaturalmedicine.com/2016/06/20/new-study-farmacy-alzheimers-aluminum-link-can-no-longer-ignored/. Accessed Jan 13, 2018.

14. Turhan S. Aluminum contents in baked meat wrapped in aluminum foil. *Meat Sci* 2006 Dec 74(4):644-647. doi: 10.1016/j.meatsci.2006.03.031.

Chapter 4: Bisphenol A, Triclosan, and 4-Nonylphenol

Bisphenol A, Triclosan, and 4-Nonylphenol are endocrine disruptors associated with these health problems: morbidity/obesity, adult onset diabetes, early puberty, reproductive system abnormalities, hormonal imbalance, thyroid disruption, ADD/ADHD, neurological development disorders, allergies, and increased cancer risk. Bisphenol A, commonly known as BPA, is a chemical used in many plastic products including bottled water, soda, and storage containers for food leftovers. BPA is commonly found in baby bottles, water bottles, food containers, beverage containers, plastic dinnerware, thermal paper receipts, medical and dental devices, eyeglass lenses, and household electronics. This harmful chemical can affect endocrine, nervous, and immune systems. Pregnant women, fetuses, infants, and children are particularly at high risk to even small amounts of exposure as it can cause problems in neurological development in fetuses and later behavioral problems in children.

BPA toxicity often lies at the root of a whole host of chronic illnesses, such as ADD/ADHD, adult onset diabetes, allergies, asthma, autoimmune disease, brain fog, chemical sensitivities, chronic bacterial, fungal, or viral infections, chronic neurological illnesses, cognitive difficulties, developmental disorders, diabetes, early puberty, fatigue, fibromyalgia, hormonal imbalances, infertility, increased risk for cancer, mood disorders, neurological developmental disorders, obesity, reproductive system disorders, and thyroid disruption.[1]

Insulin Resistance

According to recent research published in *Environmental Health Perspective*, the estrogenic properties of BPA can disrupt pancreatic beta-cell function. This is how that works: The beta cells store and release insulin, the primary hormone involved in maintaining appropriate blood-sugar levels. In the research, low-dose, long-term exposure to BPA caused a rise in insulin production that lead to insulin resistance. Other studies have indicated that elevated insulin levels are a risk factor for obesity.

Increase in Fat Cell Production

Obesity is an increase in either the number or size of fat cells, or *adipocytes*. A Japanese study found the estrogen-like effects of BPA cause *hyperplasia* (an increase in the number of fat cells) and *hypertrophy* (an enlargement of the fat cells) in laboratory mice. The effect increased with an increase in simultaneously occurring insulin production. A more recent study led by Tufts University scientists confirmed the results. Exposure to BPA increased the fat cell production in laboratory test mice whose mothers had been exposed to the chemical, despite holding other factors constant, such as calorie intake and physical activity. Those mice produced offspring that became an average of 15% heavier in adulthood.

Thyroid and Endocrine Dysfunction

BPA is an endocrine disruptor, which is an outside chemical that can mimic a natural body hormone and fool the body into over-responding, such as increasing body mass through growth hormone or stimulating insulin production when it is not needed. A 2007 study found that BPA can bind to the thyroid hormone receptor, interrupting its function. Thyroid conditions, particularly hypothyroidism, have been implicated in weight gain. Many of us have read the studies about bisphenol-A (better known as BPA), and know the chemical needs to be avoided in these products: drinking containers, baby bottles, canned foods, and thermal paper. In a 2009 CDC report, traces of BPA were found in 90% of urine samples taken from a group that was representative of the U.S. population. When a slew of new products branded "BPA-free" hit the market amid public outcry a few years back, many thought the problem solved. However, a damning new study from scientists at the University of Calgary has found that the supposed remedy, a chemical similar to BPA called bisphenol-S, may be just as bad for your health. The researchers ended the paper by recommending "a societal push to remove all bisphenols from our consumer goods."

After several states imposed bans on the use of BPA in baby bottles, many companies voluntarily removed the chemical from their products. Some, however, replaced it with an unknown alternative, later revealed to be bisphenol-S. Many consumers have assumed products were safe after reading the "BPA-free" label. But a study, published this month in the Proceedings of the National

Academy of Sciences found BPS (bisphenol-S) exposure affected prenatal neurodevelopment in zebra fish as much as BPA. This research suggests that pregnant women should be particularly mindful of their exposure to BPA and BPS throughout gestation. Additionally, the study stated that BPS itself is found in trace amounts in 81% of the U.S. population. Despite growing evidence that the chemical may be harmful to humans, the FDA reiterated its position late last year that BPA is safe to use in cans and beverage containers. The agency also rejected a complete ban in food packaging in 2012.

Triclosan is an ingredient used in many personal care products, such as deodorant, hand soap, toothpaste, mouthwash, shaving cream, cosmetics, and cleaning products to reduce or prevent the growth of bacteria.[1] Triclosan bioaccumulates in the body and is suspected to block thyroid activity, affecting metabolism and thyroid hormone signaling. Triclosan is also being added to many consumer products, such as toys, bedding, and trash bags. Exposure occurs through the use of these products in the home. Along with lots of other ingredients with hard to spell names, triclosan is an antiseptic. It's included in some products in order to kill bacteria. Now, it's understandable that people are concerned about bacteria. Good hygiene is important to keep germs and bad bacteria at bay, but antiseptics and antibacterials don't discriminate. They kill all bacteria, whether they are harmful, or not, very much like a broad-spectrum antibiotic. Bodies need bacteria to stay healthy. In fact, some bacteria can actually protect us from harmful pathogens. We are becoming aware that the microbiome within us and around us is not necessarily our enemy.

Fortunately, triclosan has been banned in the US. Studies have shown that including antibacterials in soap doesn't reduce the spread of infectious disease. There is just no need for them to be there. Furthermore, their addition may not be safe. Triclosan crosses the skin barrier. This means that it only has to come in contact with the skin and is transported transdermally to inside the body. It ends up in plasma, urine, and even breast milk. Another problem with triclosan is that in animal studies it disrupts hormones. It hasn't been deemed to be directly harmful to humans yet, but a lot of people aren't convinced it's been shown to be completely safe either.

Another serious concern with triclosan is that bacteria are adaptive. They are becoming immune to the things that used to kill them, such as penicillin. As bacteria become resistant to the triclosan and to antibiotics, the widespread use of triclosan and other antiseptics could mean that lifesaving medications become less effective.

Another endocrine system disruptor is *4-nonylphenol* because it mimics estrogen.[2,3] This toxic chemical is found in industrial detergents such as for dry cleaning and carpets, emulsifiers, wetting and foaming agents, lubricating oil additives, industrial antioxidants in plastics and rubbers, laundry and dish detergents where it is a common biodegrading product of nonylphenol ethoxylates, pesticides, and solubilizers such as in paints.[1-5] In water, 4-nonylphenol originates from the bio transformation of nonylphenol polyethoxylate (NPEO), nonionic (they have no charge) surfactants of various ethoxylate chain lengths.[1-3.] The major source of this 4-nonylphenol comes from treated wastewater effluent and land application of biosolids. Since 4-nonyphenol is hydrophobic, relatively insoluble in water, it can persist and accumulate in sediments and sludge.[3] It may take months or years to degrade in the environment.

Most exposure to 4-nonylphenol occurs through the skin. It can bind to estrogen receptors and elicit estrogenic action in vivo and in vitro.[2,3] 4-nonylphenol is reported to have a greater affinity for estrogen receptors in fish compared with humans.[3] Tests in rats for reproductive effects of 4-nonylphenol over three generations confirmed males had decreased epididymal sperm density and testicular spermatid head counts and females had increased uterus cycle length and decreased ovarian weights.[3] In breasts, 4-nonylphenol can cause cancer cells to increase in number.[4] While human exposure to 4-nonylphenol has not yet been evaluated,[1] exposure to 4-nonylphenol inhibits seed germination in some plants and growth of certain aquatic plants and algae.[5]

While there are no existing regulations for 4-nonylphenol in drinking water and the compound is not listed as a candidate for future regulatory decision-making, residues of 4-nonylphenol have been reported in river water, groundwater adjacent to a contaminated river, seawater, tap water, sediments, and fish tissues.[6]

Concentrations of 4-nonylphenol in surface waters are in the range of 0.11 to 180 micrograms per liter.[7]

Reference List

1. Genova Diagnostics. *Bishenol A profice—urine.* 2015. https://www.gdx.net/product/bisphenol-a-bpa-test-urine. Accessed Jan 5, 2018.
2. Tanghe T, Verstraete W. Adsorption of nonylphenol onto granular activated carbon. *Water, Air, and Soil Pollution* 2001 131:61-72. https://link.springer.com/article/10.1023/A:1011966914827. Accessed Jan 13, 2018.
3. Hyunook K., Guisu P, Myongjin Y, Eunjung K, Yungkook H, and Mark FC. Oxidation of nonylphenol in water using O3. *Res. J. Chem. Environ* 2007 11(2): 7-12.
4. Kim J, Korshin GV, Velichenko AB. Comparative study of electrochemical degradation and ozonation of nonylphenol. *Wat Res* 2005 39: 2527-2534.
5. Hu J, Xie G, Aizawa T. Products of aqueous chlorination of 4-nonylphenol and their estrogenic activity. *Environmental Toxicology and Chemistry* 2002 21 (10): 2034-2039.
6. Kuramitz H, Saiotoh J, Hattori T, Tanaka S. Electrochemical removal of p-nonylphenol from dilute solution using a carbon fiber anode. *Wat Res* 2002 36: 3323-3329.
7. Yu Z. *Analysis of selected pharmaceuticals and endocrine disrupting compounds and their removal by granular activated carbon in drinking water treatment.* Doctoral dissertation, the University of Waterloo, Ontario, Canada. 2002.
8. Cox C. Nonyl phenol and related chemicals. *Journal of Pesticide Reform* 1996 16 (1).

The chemicals discussed above are often found in drinking water and in the water in which we bathe, shower, swim, and wash clothes. One of the frequent recommendations I make to my patients who have chronic health problems or just want to be more preventative in their approach to health is to acquire a drinking water filtration system that removes all these toxins from their drinking water and laundry and house systems so that the amounts coming in transdermal contact with their bodies is reduced. In a later chapter, I suggest some of these systems.

The following companies produce triclosan-free products.
Big Green Smile for liquid soaps
Faith in Nature for bar soaps
Green People for toothpaste.

Chapter 5: Chlorinated Pesticides

DDT is probably the best-known chlorinated pesticide. Other chlorinated pesticides include methoxychlor, aldrin, dieldrin, chlordane, toxaphene, endrin, heptachlor, and lindane (gamma isomer of benzene hexachloride (BHC).[1] While the use of these pesticides is mostly banned in the U.S., they continue to be a health threat because they persist in the environment, are bioaccumulative, and difficult to excrete from the body.[2] Genova Diagnostics finds that 98% of those tested have been identified with having chlorinated pesticides in their systems.[3]

Discovered in 1939 by Swiss Chemist Paul Muller, DDT was considered a miracle for three reasons: It was toxic to a wide range of insects and initially appeared to have low toxicity to mammals, did not break down rapidly in the environment, and did not wash away by rain. It was used for virtually everything, including delousing soldiers and children. However, the very qualities that made it a wonder pesticide are also why this pesticide and others like it are so dangerous: They persist and concentrations increase up the food chain. While DDT hasn't been used in the U.S. since 1972, it and other chlorinated pesticides still exists in the environment, being absorbed by plant and animal life[4] and present in some U.S. water supplies.[5] Chlorinated pesticides concentrate in the brain and fat tissue.

The Stockholm Convention on Persistent Organic Pollutants banning the use of all chlorinated pesticides went into effect in 2004 with 152 countries participating. The U.S., however, is not participating in this ban.[5] Certain developing nations with a prevalence of malaria have an exemption because DDT is still the cheapest and most effective pesticide against mosquitos. While originally it was believed that DDT, and by analogy other chlorinated pesticides, was not toxic to mammals, subsequent studies have proven that assumption false. In experimental animals, DDT has caused chronic effects on the nervous system, liver, kidneys, adrenal glands, and immune systems. Experiments with animals also found that DDT causes reproductive effects, impairs learning rates in offspring, and increases tumor production in several organs.[6] Because DDT is airborne, it has been found in such faraway places as the Arctic, in the blubber of sperm whales, and the muscles of Antarctic penguins.

One study did find a suggested link between DDT levels and pancreatic cancer in humans.[6] Compare the results of the animal studies to the 98% percentage of humans found chlorinated pesticides.[3] A potential danger lies with pesticides as endocrine disrupters as has been shown in wildlife exposed to these pesticides.[7]

Although unlikely in most circumstances, acute chlorinated pesticide toxicity leads to initial euphoria with auditory or visual hallucinations and perceptual disturbances, seizures, and agitation, lethargy, or unconsciousness. Additional symptoms affect the pulmonary system--coughing and shortness of breath, the dermis--skin rash, the gastrointestinal system--nausea, vomiting, diarrhea, and abdominal pain, and the nervous system—headache, dizziness, or paresthesia of the face. Ingesting a chlorinated pesticide creates nausea and vomiting, confusion, tremors, myocionus, coma, seizures respiratory distress or failure, and an unusual turpentine odor.

If the chlorinated pesticide is absorbed through the skin, there may be ear, nose, and throat irritation, blurred vision, coughing, acute lung injury, and dermatitis. Chronic exposure brings on anorexia, hepatoxicity, renal toxicity, central nervous system disturbances, and skin irritation.[8] The persistence of these chlorinated pesticides are the primary reason there are still health concerns. They pose a health danger because they accumulate in the body, primarily in the brain and fatty tissue.

The Chlorinated Pesticides Profile Test from Genova Diagnostics can help to identify when a patient has been exposed to certain pesticides and insecticides and how high the levels are. This panel looks at the most commonly found chlorinated pesticides, which have national reference ranges that have been documented to cause adverse health problems. Levels are given both in parts per million (PPM) and as lipid-adjusted amounts so the clinician can best estimate the total body burden of these compounds. Chlorinated pesticides can also be detected in the GPL-Tox: Toxic Non-Metal Chemical Profile from Great Plains Laboratory.

Because of the high rate of prevalence of chlorinated pesticides in the population I routinely evaluate the body burden in patients who have any of the above symptoms. Properly washing of food is essential. Much of the poisoning is occurring through the drinking water and transdermally when bathing and showering. Proper filtration with the new 401 rating is required to remove these environmental toxins from the drinking water.

Reference List

1. Michigan Department of Natural Resources. *DDT and other chlorinated hydrocarbon pesticides.* http://www.michigan.gov/dnr/0,4570,7-153-10370_12150_12220-26633--,00.html. 2018. Accessed Jan 19, 2018.
2. Crinnion WJ. Chlorinated pesticides: threats to health and importance of detection. *Altern Med Rev* 2009 Dec;14(4):347-59.
3. Genova Diagnostics. *Chlorinated pesticides profile-serum.* https://www.gdx.net/product/chlorinated-pesticides-test-serum. 2015. Accessed Jan 19, 2018.
4. Muir P. *A. history of pesticide use.* Oct 22, 2012. http://people.oregonstate.edu/~muirp/pesthist.htm. Accessed Jan 19, 2018.
5. Trautman NM, Porter KS, Wagenet RJ. Pesticides: health effects in drinking water. *Pesticide Safety Education Program.* http://psep.cce.cornell.edu/facts-slides-self/facts/pes-heef-grw85.aspx. 2012. Accessed Jan 20, 2018.
6. *Status of ratification.* Stockholm Convention. http://chm.pops.int/Countries/StatusofRatifications/PartiesandSignatoires/tabid/4500/Default.aspx. 2008. Accessed Jan 19, 2018.
7. Wong ML. Organochlorine pesticide toxicity. *Medscape.* Dec 29, 2015. https://emedicine.medscape.com/article/815051-overview. Accessed Jan 19, 2018.
8. Extension Toxicology Network. *DDT (dichlorodiphenyltichloroethane).* http://pmep.cce.cornell.edu/profiles/extoxnet/carbaryl-dicrotophos/ddt-ext.html.
9. Mnif W, Hassine AIH, Bouaziz A, Bartiegi A, Thomas O, Roig B. Effect of endocrine disrupter pesticides: a review.

Ent J Environ Res Public Health 2011, Jun;8(6):2265-2303.
doi: 10.3390/ijerph8062265.

Chapter 6: Polychlorinated Biphenyls (PCBs)

Between 1881 and 1914, enough PCBs were released into the environment worldwide that PCBs can still be found in certain species of birds. PCBs were used as lubricants and coolants in transformers, capacitors, and electronic equipment because of a high resistance to heat. Like chlorinated pesticides, they persist and bio-accumulate in animals and humans. The U.S. Congress banned their use in 1979, and the Stockholm Convention on Persistent Organic Pollutants banned their use in 2001. Despite the ban, PCBs can be found in old transformers and continue to leach into soil and groundwater from hazardous waste sites and landfills.[1]

Here is what happens when PCBs enter the body. Like other toxins, they are absorbed by and stored in fat cells. Since PCBs are not water-soluble, they are not excreted from the body and accumulate over a person's lifetime, increasing that person's body burden of PCBs. In adults, a heavy burden of PCBs over time can cause impairments in the brain, nervous system, endocrine system, and immune system and may cause fertility issues. An accumulation of PCBs affects children more than adults. PCBs can be passed to children through the placenta and breastfeeding. A Michigan study of mothers who had eaten PCB contaminated fish found that infants born to those with the greatest consumption of the contaminated fish had weaker reflexes, greater motor immaturity, and a pronounced startle response. These perinatal effects persisted with these same children so that by age 4 they showed depressed weight gain and responsiveness and reduced performance on visual recognition-memory tests. Even after 11 years, these same children were 3 times more likely to have low full-scale verbal IQ scores, twice as likely to be lagging in reading comprehension, and more likely to have difficulty paying attention than children without this exposure. Children born to women who worked with PCBs in factories showed decreased birth weight and a significant decrease in gestational age with increasing exposure to PCBs.[2]

PCB exposure in early childhood may result in a lowered immune response. One study found that this early exposure created a greater risk for development of diphtheria and tetanus later in life even if the child has been immunized.[3] Of course, you now know that these vaccines contain mercury and/or aluminum, so these children are getting a toxic double whammy. A compromised immune system can lead to allergies, sensitivities, and chronic infections in children.

Persistence of PCBs in the environment continues to create health problems. As with other toxins, the PCBs bio-accumulate, moving up the food chain to fish, meat, and dairy products, especially from areas of the country considered contaminated. Because PCBs are no longer manufactured or widely used today, there are relatively few ways that people can be exposed to concentrated PCBs. Consequently, the most common exposure comes from food, surface soils, drinking and ground water, indoor air, and industrial accidents.

- **Food:** PCBs in food are probably the single most significant source of exposure for people. PCBs can be highly concentrated in the fish of waters contaminated with even low levels of PCBs. Predator fish at the top of the food chain, as well as bottom feeding fish, tend to contain the highest PCB levels in those waters. PCBs have been found in shellfish, beef, butter, and milk. For the beef, butter, and milk, choose organic to avoid this contamination.[4]
- **Surface Soils:** PCBs are among the second most likely group of chemicals requiring clean up in soils.[5] The health hazard is related to the potential for people to swallow small amounts of the soil and for the soils to runoff to lakes and rivers and concentrate in fish and other wildlife.[5]
- **Drinking Water and Groundwater:** It is a rare occurrence for PCBs to be found in groundwater. However, it is possible for oil containing PCBs in submersible pumps in private wells to leak.[6] The EPA goal for drinking water is zero and the enforceable levels in microliters for PCBs in public water supplies is 0.0005ppm (parts per million).[7] Check reports on your own municipal water supply.
- **Indoor Air:** Older fluorescent lights found in schools, offices, and homes may still contain transformers or

ballasts that contain PCBs. If the ballasts fail, PCBs can leak out and contaminate exposed surfaces and the air.[8]

- **In the Workplace:** Industrial accidents have been responsible for most cases of acute PCB poisoning in humans. Firefighters and cleanup crews responding to electrical system fires and hazardous waste accidents also may be exposed to PCBs.

While the likelihood of PCB exposure has been reduced since its ban, here are some symptoms of exposure to high levels of PCBs.

- Severe acne
- Rash
- Eye irritation
- Liver damage
- Weakened immune system
- Chemical sensitivity
- Allergies
- Obesity
- Fatigue
- Certain cancers
- Developmental disorders[9]

To reiterate the potential dangers from PCB exposure, data strongly suggest that PCBs are probable human carcinogens.[2,9] Studies in animals and humans suggest that long term exposure to PCBs can suppress the immune system.[2] PCBs have been demonstrated to exert effects on thyroid hormone levels in animals and humans.[2,10, 11, 12] Thyroid hormone levels are critical for normal growth and development. Alterations in thyroid hormone levels may have significant implications for health.

These are some suggested guidelines to prevent PCB exposure.

- Pregnant mothers, women who plan to become pregnant, children and nursing mothers should limit their consumption of sport-caught fish from waters contaminated with PCBs.
- If you live near a hazardous waste facility, make sure children do not play directly in the soil. Practice good

hygiene habits. Wash children's hands and faces after playing and before eating. Do not let them eat the dirt.

- If any member of the household works with old electrical equipment including transformers be sure that the equipment is properly maintained and the area is well ventilated.

The Polychlorinated Biphenyls (PCBs) Profile through blood serum testing from Genova Laboratories can help identify which of the most toxic PCBs you may have been exposed to and your body burden. The most commonly found PCBs that have national reference ranges that have been documented to cause adverse health problems are measured. Levels are given both in parts per million (PPM) and as lipid-adjusted amounts so the clinician can best estimate the total body burden of these compounds.[13]

Polychlorinated biphenyl testing can help you determine the extent of this PCB burden. PCBs can also be evaluated through the urine in the GPL-Tox Panel through Great Plains Laboratories.[14] I recommend PCBs evaluation for any woman who is considering getting pregnant. It is important to reduce the body burden of PCBs to have a healthy baby.

Reference List

1. *Polychlorinated biphenyl (PCB) wastes: background on PCBS and their impacts.* University Library, University of Illinois at Urbana-Champaign. http://guides.library.illinois.edu/c.php?g=348351&p=2347270. 2017. Accessed Jan 20, 2018.
2. Agency for Toxic Substance & Disease Registry. *Polychlorinated biphenyls (PCBs) toxicity: what are adverse health effects of PCB exposure?* Aug 9, 2016. https://www.atsdr.cdc.gov/csem/csem.asp?csem=30&po=10. Accessed Jan 25, 2018.
3. Barret J. Diminished protection?: early childhood PCB exposure and reduced immune response to vaccinations. *Environ Health Perspect* 210 Oct; 118(10):A4-45. doi: 10.1289/ehp.118-a445a.
4. Fitzpatrick T. PCBs (polychlorinated biphenyls) are in the foods you love. *Environ, Chem & Haz News, Car & Res.*

environmentalchemistry.com. Jan 31, 2006. Accessed Jan 25, 2018.

5. Cunningham SD, Anderson TA, Schwab AP, Hsu FC. *Phytoremediation of soils contaminated with organic pollutants.* https://s3.amazonaws.com/academia.edu.documents/4427929 4/Phytoremediation_of_Soils_Contaminated_w20160331- 11761- ll9jaf.pdf?AWSAccessKeyId=AKIAIWOWYYGZ2Y53UL3 A&Expires=1517004939&Signature=PJDe%2Bl3VoIHEd2 UdMAdqcu9QG7c%3D&response-content- disposition=inline%3B%20filename%3DPhytoremediation_ of_Soils_Contaminated_w.pdf. Sep 11, 2015. Accessed Jan 26, 2018.

6. Carbon Country Groundwater Guardians. *How to clean out a private well—suspected of PCB oil contamination from well pump.* http://carbonwaters.org/2014/08/how-to-clean-out-a- private-well-suspected-of-pcb-oil-contamination-from-well- pump/. 2018. Accessed Jan 25, 2018.

7. Agency for Toxic Substance & Disease Registry. Polycholorinated biphenyls (PCBs) toxicity: what standards and regulations exist for PCB exposure? *Environ Health Ed.* Aug 9, 2016. https://www.atsdr.cdc.gov/csem/csem.asp?csem=30&po=8.. Accessed Jan 25, 2018.

8. United States Environmental Protection Agency. Polychlorinated biphenyl (PCB)—containing florescent light ballasts (FLBs) in school buildings. *Polychlorinated Biphenyl.* Jan 18, 2018. https://www.epa.gov/pcbs/polychlorinated-biphenyl-pcb- containing-fluorescent-light-ballasts-flbs-school-buildings. Accessed Jan 25, 2018.

9. What are the human health effects of PCBs?. *Clearwater News & Bulletins.* http://www.clearwater.org/news/pcbhealth.html. Accessed Jan 25, 2018.

10. Schell LM, Gallo MV, Denham M, Ravenscroft J, DeCaprio A, Carpenter DO. Relationship of thyroid levels of polychlorinated biphenyls, lead, *p, p'*-DDE, and other

---

toxicants in Akwesasne Mohawk youth. *Environ Health Perspect* 2008 Jun; 116(6):806-813. doi: 10.1289/ehp.10490.

11. Gauger KJ, Kato Y, Haraguchi K, et al. Polychlorinated biphenyls (PCBs) exert thyroid hormone-like effects in the fetal rat brain but do not bind to thyroid hormone receptors. *Environ Health Percept* 2004 Apr; 112(5):516-523. https://www.ncbi.nlm.nih.gov/pmc/articles/PMC2430238/. Accessed Jan 25, 2018.

12. Gauger KJ. *The effects of polychlorinated biphenyls on thyroid hormone-mediated action in vivo and invitro.* Dissertation, University of Massachusetts Amherst, AAI3206211. 2006.

13. Genova Diagnostics. https://www.gdx.net/. 2015. Accessed Jan 25, 2018.

14. Great Plains Laboratory, Inc. https://www.greatplainslaboratory.com/. Accessed Jan 25, 2018.

Chapter 7: Phthalates and Parabens

Phthalates

Plasticizers or specifically *phthalates* are now considered the number one pollutant in the human body. Phthalates make plastics soft and pliable. They also dissolve fragrance in perfumes. Research has shown that exposure to phthalates can lead to chronic health problems, including cancer, liver toxicity, reproductive toxicity, problems with the development of puberty, and more. Phthalates are over 10,000 to 1,000,000 times higher in human bodies than any other toxins found in EPA studies.[1]

Phthalates are found in a wide range of every day products: plastic, plastic food containers, plastic toys, furniture, car interiors, blood IV bags, vinyl flooring, adhesives, fragrances, detergents, and air fresheners.[2] While there are no human studies documenting the harm done by phthalates, animal studies are suggestive.[3] Phthalates may be particularly dangerous for pregnant women.

- Phthalates can damage the chemistry of fatty acid DHA (docosahexaenoic acid). DHA is part of polyunsaturated fatty acids in fish oil. This is the fundamental chemistry necessary for making every cell lining or membrane. These fatty acids are the foundation for brain health including memory and recall. Low DHA can lead to chronic inflammation. The results of one study with rats, for instance, suggest that phthalate may alter placental essential fatty acid homeostasis, thereby potentially resulting in abnormal fetal development. This happens because the phthalate lowers DHA.[4] These same results were verified by a 2008 study with a suggestion that it leads to fetal toxicity.[5]

- Phthalates induces a zinc deficiency during pregnancy and congenital malformations[6] and testicular atrophy in adult male rats.[7] Zinc deficiency compromises the metabolism of vitamins A and B-6, which, in turn, can contribute to indigestion, depression, heart disease, cancer, diabetes, and accelerated aging. Low zinc can lead to chronic inflammation.[8]

- Phthalates damages pancreas beta cells leading to diabetes, insulin resistance, and metabolic syndrome X. Exposure to this chemical contaminant prenatally and during adolescence can increase this risk.[9]

- Phthalates has been found to lower the body's ability for sulfation.[10] Sulfation is an essential detoxification process that needs adequate glutathione, one of the three most powerful inherent anti-oxidants in the body. This means that you are no longer able to effectively detoxify like you should. This in turn can lead to many chronic illnesses and diseases.

- Phthalates are endocrine disruptors.[11, 12, 13] They damage hormone function, especially thyroid and testosterone. This is a contributing factor to the epidemic of hypothyroidism and low testosterone in this country and Northern Europe.

- Phthalates may cause high cholesterol[14] while at the same time inhibit the production of the neurotransmitters of the brain.[15]

- Phthalates can damage the body's ability to make catalase. Catalase is one of the three most powerful inherent anti-oxidants in the body. Catalase is absolutely essential for scavenging the hydrogen peroxide that cancer cells make to allow them to metastasize and spread throughout the body. Lack of catalase is one reason why many cancers briefly seem to be in remission after treatments, only to resurface months or years later with lethal consequences. This phenomenon has been recorded in carp[16] and rats[17.]

Reference List

1. Grisanti R. 7 ways plastics damage the body. *Functional Medicine University.* https://www.functionalmedicineuniversity.com/public/919.cf m. 2018. Accessed Jan 25, 2018.

2. *Phthalates: The everywhere chemical.*
   https://www.niehs.nih.gov/research/supported/assets/docs/j_q
   /phthalates_the_everywhere_chemical_handout_508.pdf.
   Accessed Jan 25, 2018.
3. Center for Disease Control and Prevention. *Phthaltes fact sheet.*
   https://www.cdc.gov/biomonitoring/Phthalates_FactSheet.ht
   ml. Apr 7, 2017. Accessed Jan 25, 2018.
4. Xu Y, Cook TJ, Knipp GT. Effects of di-(2ethyhexyl)-
   phthalate (DEHP) and its metabolites on fatty acid
   homeostasis in rat placental HRP-trophoblast cells. *Toxicol
   Sci* 2005, Apr; 84(2): 287-300.
   https://www.ncbi.nlm.nih.gov/pubmed/15647598. Accessed
   Jan 26, 2018.
5. Xu Y, Agrawai S, Cook TJ, Knipp GT. Maternal di-(2
   ethylhexyl)-phthalate exposure influences essential fatty acid
   homeostasis in rat placenta. *Placenta* 2008, Nov, 29(11):
   962-969. doi: 10.1016/j.placenta.2008.08.011.
6. Peters JM, Taubeneck JM, Keen CL, Gonzalez FJ. Di-(2-
   ethyhexyl)-phthlate induces a functional zinc deficiency
   during pregnancy and teratogenesis that is independent of
   peroxisome proliferator-activated receptor-alpha. *Teratology*
   1997, Nov; 56(5): 311-6.
   https://www.ncbi.nlm.nih.gov/pubmed/9451755. Accessed
   Jan 26, 2018.
7. Agarwal DK, Eustis S, Lamb IV JC, Jameson CW, Kluwe
   WM. Influence of dietary zinc on di(2-ethylhexyl)phthalate-
   induced testicular atrophy and zinc depletion in adult rats.
   Tox and App Pharma 1986 Jun 15; 84(1): 12-24. doi:
   10.1016/0041-008X(86)90412-6.
8. Gammoh NZ, Rink L. Zinc in infection and inflammation.
   Nutrients 2017 Jun; 9(6): 624. doi: 0.3390/nu9060624.
9. Fabricio G, Malta A, Chango A, Cezar de Freitas Mathias P.
   Environmental contaminants and pancreatic beta cells. *J Clin
   Res Pediatr Endocrinol* 2016 Sep; 8(3): 257-263. doi:
   10.4274/jcrpe.2812.
10. Harris RM, Waring RH. Potential impact of diet and
    environmental chemicals on steroid metabolism and drug

detoxification. *Curr Drug Metab* 2008 May; 9(4): 269-275(7). doi: 10.2174/138920008784220637.

11. Miodovnik A, Engel SM, Zhu C, et al. Endocrine disruptors and social impairment. *NeuroTox* 2011 Mar; 32(2): 261-267. doi: 10.1016/j.neuro.2010.12.009.

12. Casal-Casas C, Desvergne B. Endocrine disruptors: from endocrine to metabolic disruption. *Ann Rev Physiol* 2011 Mar; 73: 135-162. doi: 10.1146/annurev-physiol-012110-142200.

13. Dodson RF, Nishioka M, Standley LJ, Perovich LJ, Brody JG, Rudel RA. Endocrine disruptors and asthma-association chemicals in consumer products. *Environ Health Perspect* 2012 Jul; 120(7): 935-943. doi: 10.1289/ehp.1104052.

14. Moody DE, Reddy JK. Serum triglyceride and cholesterol contents in male rats receiving diets containing plasticizers and analogues of the ester 2-ethylhexonal. *Toxicology Letters* 10 (4); 1982: 379-383. doi:10.1016/0378-4274(82)90233-8.

15. Carbone S, Szwarcfarb B, Ponzo O, et.al. Impact of gestational and lactational phthalate exposure on hypothalamic content of amino acid neurotransmitters and FSH secretion in peripubertal male rats. *NeuroToxicology* 31(6); 2010: 747-751. doi: 10.1016/j.neuro.2010.06.006.

16. Zhao X, Gao Y, Mingliang Q. Toxicity of phthalate esters exposure to carp (Cyprinus carpio) and antioxidant response by biomarker. *Ecotoxicology* 2014; 23(4): 628-632. doi: 10.1007/s10646-014-1194-x.

17. Rusyn I, Peter JM, Cunningham ML. Effects of DEHP in the liver: modes of action and species-specific differences. *Crit Rev Toxic* 2006 May; 36(5): 459-479. doi: 10.1080/10408440600779065.

Parabens

Parabens are additives to keep mold and fungi from growing in almost every personal care product use today. Products that contain parabens are cosmetics, lotions, soaps, shampoos, sunscreens, moisturizers, shaving gels, and toothpaste, to name a few. Parabens are used commonly as a preservative, and they easily penetrate the skin. The European Commission on Endocrine Disruption lists parabens as a category 1 substance, shown to be an endocrine disruptor. The ability of parabens to penetrate human skin intact without breaking down and to be absorbed systemically has been demonstrated through studies and extensively documented.[1] Parabens go by the following names: Methylparaben, butylparaben, propylparaben, isobutylparaben, ethylparaben, polyparaben and isobutylparaben.[2]

Parabens has been detected in human tissue, and its presence in breast tissue of patients with breast cancer is particularly troubling.[3] Additionally, there is some concern about the role of parabens with male reproductive functions and in melanoma.[1]

The following is a list in alphabetic order of paraben-free products with their web addresses.

Aurelia Probiotic Skincare
    http://www.aureliaskincare.com/
Aromatherapy Associates
    http://www.aromatherapyassociates.com/
Balance Me
    https://www.balanceme.co.uk/
BareMinerals
    http://bareminerals.co.uk/
BEAUBRONZ
    http://www.beaubronz.co.uk/
Bee Good Skincare
    http://beegood.co.uk/
Bionsen Deodorant
    http://www.bionsen.co.uk/
Bodhi & Birch
    https://www.bodhiandbirch.com
Boots Botanics
    http://www.boots.com/en/Botanics/
Burt's Bees
    http://www.burtsbees.co.uk/
Butter London
    http://www.butterlondon.com/
COWSHED
    http://www.cowshedonline.com/
Dr Hauschka
    http://www.drhauschka.co.uk/home
Figs & Rouge

http://www.figsandrouge.com/
Good Things
    http://www.goodthingsbeauty.com/
Green People
    http://www.greenpeople.co.uk/
Hearts and Homespun
    http://www.heartsandhomespun.com/
Hourglass Cosmetics
    http://hourglasscosmetics.com/
Ila
    http://www.ila-spa.com/shop
Inika Cosmetics
    http://inikacosmetics.co.uk/
Just Soaps Of The Earth
    http://www.justsoapsoftheearth.co.uk/
Karin Herzog
    http://www.karinherzog.co.uk/
Kiss My Face
    https://www.kissmyface.com/
Korres
    http://www.korres.com/
Lavera
    http://www.pravera.co.uk/lavera-natural-cosmetics
Lily Lolo Mineral Cosmetics
    http://www.lilylolo.co.uk/
Living Nature
    http://www.livingnature.com/
Lulu and Boo Organics
    http://www.luluandboo.com/
Mandara Spa
    http://www.timetospa.co.uk/mandara-spa/
Marshmallow Blends
http://www.marshmallowblends.co.uk/
Melvita
    http://uk.melvita.com/
Mill Creek Botanicals
    https://millcreekbotanicals.com
Myroo Skincare
    http://www.myroo.co.uk/

Neal's Yard Remedies
   http://www.nealsyardremedies.com/
NEOM
   http://neomorganics.com/
NUDE Skincare
   http://www.nudeskincare.com/
Nuxe
   https://uk.nuxe.com
Organic Surge
   http://www.organicsurge.com
Pai Skincare
   http://www.paiskincare.com
Palm and Sole
   http://www.palm-and-sole.com
Pinks Boutique
   http://www.pinksboutique.com/
Pure Lochside
   http://www.purelochside.com/
Pure Thoughts
   http://www.purethoughts.co.uk/
Ren Skincare
   http://www.renskincare.com/
RMS Beauty
   http://www.beingcontent.com/filter/brand/rms-
beauty.html
Sam Pure MakeUp
   http://www.sampure.co.uk/
Savar
   http://www.savaronline.co.uk/
Soothing Showers
   http://www.soothingshowers.com/
Susan Posnick Cosmetics
   http://www.susanposnick.com/
Weleda
   http://www.weleda.co.uk/
Yes To
   http://www.yestocarrots.com/find-a-store-uk.html
Youngblood Mineral Cosmetics
   http://ybskin.co.uk/

Phthalates and Parabens Profile

When it comes to phthalates and parabens, I feel it is better to err on the side of caution with these chemicals. The Phthalates and Parabens Profile can help to identify everyday exposure to toxins from the use of personal care products and plastic food containers. This profile is a great option if you're experiencing prolonged chronic health problems or to determine if your body is detoxifying properly. Environmental toxins should be evaluated as a first step to help patients get back on the road to wellness.[9] This urine test is available from Genova Diagnostics[4] and it also available through the GPL-Tox—Toxic Non-Metal Chemical Profile from Great Plains Laboratory.[5] Reduction of phthalates and parabens in the body is essential for a healthy hormone system.

Reference List

1. Darbre PD, Harvey PW. Paraben esters: review of recent studies of endocrine toxicity, absorption, esterase and human exposure, and discussion of health risks. *J Appl Toxicol* 2008 Jul: 28(5): 561-78. doi: 10.1002/jat.1358.
2. Chemcalland 21. *Parabens (methy, ethyl, propyl, butyl).* http://www.chemicalland21.com/lifescience/foco/PARABEN S/(METHYL, ETHYL, PROPYL, 0BUTYL).htm. Accessed Jan 27, 2018.
3. Kirchhof MG, deGannes JC. The health controversies of parabens. *Skin Therap Lett* 2013 Feb; 18(2): 5-7. https://www.ncbi.nlm.nih.gov/pubmed/23508773. Accessed Jan 27, 2018.
4. Genova Diagnostics. 2015. https://www.gdx.net/. Accessed Jan 27, 2018.
5. The Great Plains Laboratory, Inc. https://www.greatplainslaboratory.com/. Accessed Jan 27, 2018.

Chapter 8: Volatile Solvents

Volatile solvents are routinely used in industrial processes to manufacture consumer products. A solvent is a liquid or gas used to dissolve a solid, liquid, or gas to create a new solution. Each year, annual production of these solvents numbers in the tens of billions of pounds in the United States. Chemicals can enter the body through three major pathways: breathing, touching, or swallowing. Air and water pollution are common routes of exposure in homes and workplaces. We are also exposed by inhalation or ingestion of car exhaust, paints, glues, adhesives, and lacquer thinners.

These volatile solvents are used in large numbers to produce items in our homes, such as furniture, building materials, paint, shoes, cleaning and degreasing agents, inks, pharmaceuticals, and as additives to gasoline. For those living and working in urban areas, the exposure to this class of compounds goes on twenty-four hours a day. Glue is a volatile solvent that is sometimes abused.

Solvents are very damaging to bone marrow and have been associated with many of the bone marrow cancers[1,3] as well as anemia[1-3] and thrombocytopenia.[4] They are also associated with immune disorders,[5] including autoimmunity, chronic neurologic problems, and infertility.[6] Overexposure or chronic exposure to volatile solvents damages the central nervous system and causes chemical-driven liver and kidney damage.[7] Benzene, in particular, has a severe toxic effect on the hematological system and is a recognized human carcinogen. Other solvents contribute to atrophy of skeletal muscles,[8] loss of coordination,[8,9] vision problems,[8] and depression of the central nervous system.[8,9]

Symptoms of Solvent Exposure[10,11]

- Aplastic anemia (low blood cells in bone marrow)
- Atrophy of skeletal muscles
- B-cell malignancies
- Blood dyscrasias (unspecified blood disorder)
- Bone marrow damage
- Cancer
- Chemical bronchitis
- Chromosomal aberrations
- Cognitive disorders

- Conjunctivitis
- Corneal erosion
- Defatting dermatitis
- Dermatitis
- Erectile dysfunction
- Erythema (redness due to capillary congestion)
- Fatigue
- Headaches
- Hemolysis
- Hepatomegaly (enlarged liver)
- Infertility
- Irritation of eyes and nose
- Irritation of mucous membranes
- Keratitis (cornea inflammation)
- Leukemia
- Muscular weakness
- Nausea
- Paresthesia
- Parkinsonism
- Polyneuropathy (neurological disorder)
- Pulmonary edema (fluid in lungs)
- Renal damage
- Skin irritation
-

Whether or not a person has health effects after breathing in volatile organic compounds (VOCs) depends on three factors.

1. The toxicity of the chemical (the amount of harm that can be caused by contact with the chemical).
2. How much of the chemical is in the air.
3. How long and how often the air is breathed.

Differences in age, health condition, gender and exposure to other chemicals also can affect whether or not a person experiences health effects. Short-term exposure to high levels of some VOCs can cause headaches, dizziness, light-headedness, drowsiness, nausea, and eye and respiratory irritation.[10] These effects usually go away after the exposure stops.

You can avoid exposure to many of these chemicals by using a mask in a well-ventilated area. However, it is possible that you are unaware of continued exposure in your home from carpet, furniture, vinyl flooring, shower curtains, mattresses, and the like. Using the right kind of air filtration unit (see Chapter 15: Air Pollution Solutions) can markedly reduce exposure.

The Volatile Solvents Profile is a whole blood test that can help identify a patient's prolonged exposure to the most commonly found volatile solvents that have been shown to cause serious health problems. This test is available through Genova Diagnostics. Volatile Solvents[11] can also be evaluated through Great Plains Laboratory through urine in the GPL-Tox: Toxic Non-Metal Chemical Profile.[12]

Reference List

1. Greenberg MI. *Occupational, Industrial, and Environmental Toxicology.* Philadelphia, PA: Mosby; 1991.
2. Vigilani EC. Leukemia associated with benzene exposure. *Annals of the New York Academy of Sciences* May 1976; 271: 143-151. doi: 10.1111/j.1749-6632. 1976.tb23103.x.
3. Snyder R. The benzene problem in historical perspective. *Fundamental and Applied Toxicology* Oct 1984; 4 (5): 692-699. doi: 10.1016/0272-0590(84)90090-3.
4. Aksoy M, Dinçol, Akgün T, Erdim S, Dinçol G. Haematological effects of chronic benzene poisoning in 217 workers. *Br J Ind Med* 1971 Jul; 28(3): 296-302. https://www.ncbi.nlm.nih.gov/pmc/articles/PMC1069505/. Accessed Feb 8, 2018.
5. Dung X, Chen X, Shien L, Chen C, Tingzhang Y. Effect of benzene on immunity function of exposed workers. *Journal of Hunan Medical University* 1994; 3. http://en.cnki.com.cn/Article_en/CJFDTOTAL-HNYK403.010.htm. Accessed Feb 8, 2018.
6. Bahadar H, Mostafalou S, Abdollahi M. Current understandings and perspectives on non-cancer health effects of benzene: a global concern. *Toxicology and Applied Pharmacology* 15 Apr 2015; 276(2): 83-94. doi: 10.1016/j.taap.2014.02.012.
7. Rana SV, Verma Y. Biochemical toxicity of benzene. *Journal of Environmental Biology* 1 Apr 2005; 26(2): 157-168.

8. Aungudornpukdee P, Vichit-Vadakan N. Risk factors affecting visual-motor deficit among children residing near a petrochemical industrial estate. *Nepal Med Coll J* 2009; 11(4): 241-246.

9. Jovanovic J, Jovanovic M. Neurotoxic effects of organic solvents among workers in paint and lacquer manufacturing industry [ABSTRACT]. *Med Pregi* Jan-Feb 2004; 57 (1-2): 22-25. https://www.ncbi.nlm.nih.gov/pubmed/15327185. Accessed Feb 8, 2018.

10. United States Environmental Protection Agency. *Volatile organic compounds' impact on indoor air quality.* Nov 16, 2017. https://www.epa.gov/indoor-air-quality-iaq/volatile-organic-compounds-impact-indoor-air-quality. Accessed Feb 8, 2018.

11. Genova Diagnostics. *Volatile Solvents Profile—Whole Blood.* 2015. https://www.gdx.net/product/volatile-solvents-test-blood. Accessed Feb 8, 2018.

12. The Great Plains Laboratory, Inc. GPL-Tox: toxic non-metal chemical profile. https://www.greatplainslaboratory.com/gpl-tox/. Accessed Feb 9, 2018.

Chapter 9: Glyphosate

Unless you are eating organic foods and drinking properly filtered water, you are undoubtedly being exposed to glyphosate, an herbicide patented as an antibiotic. All the leaders in natural health care that I read or follow have posted a blog on their websites and podcasts or written in their books about the dangers associated with the use of glyphosate in the food supply. William Shaw and Matthew Pratt-Hyatt, director and associate director of the Great Plains Laboratory, Inc., have outline the numerous and outstanding health risks.[1] I am indebted to them for much of the following information.

Glyphosate is the most widely produced herbicide globally, the primary toxic chemical in Roundup™, and a broad-spectrum herbicide used in more than 700 different products from agriculture and forestry to home use. Introduced in the 1970s, glyphosate works by targeting the enzymes that produce the amino acids tyrosine, tryptophan, and phenylalanine. Bacteria, algae, and fungi produce the same amino acids via the same pathway, called the Shikimate Pathway. Since humans lack this pathway, the manufacturers of glyphosate claim that this chemical is non-toxic to humans. Unfortunately, humans eat plants that have been treated with the compound and meat from animals fed plants contaminated with it.

After the introduction of genetically modified (GMO) and glyphosate-resistant crops that grow well in the presence of this compound in the soil, the use of glyphosate grew. Polyoxyethyleneamine (POEA), the surfactant often added to glyphosate, is more toxic than glyphosate itself, thereby increasing the toxicity.[2] In 2014, Canada and the U.S. approved the use of an herbicide product containing 2, 4-dichlorophenoxyacetic acid (2, 4-d), a key component of Agent Orange,[3] and glyphosate named Enlist Duo™ for use on soybeans and maize genetically modified to be resistant to both compounds.

Glyphosate and Chronic Health Conditions

According to one group of researchers, "Roundup was among the most toxic herbicides and insecticides tested."[4] Another study implicates glyphosate as the most important culprit in celiac disease.[5] Because glyphosate has been found to deplete manganese,

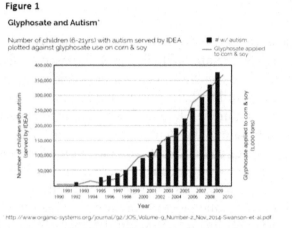

Figure 1

Glyphosate and Autism*

Number of children (6-21yrs) with autism served by IDEA plotted against glyphosate use on corn & soy

■ # w/ autism
— Glyphosate applied to corn & soy

http://www.organic-systems.org/journal/92/JOS_Volume-9_Number-2_Nov_2014-Swanson-et-al.pdf

Figure 1 used with permission of Shaw & Pratt-Hyatt, 2017.

there is a resulting plethora of neurological diseases and pathologies—autism, Alzheimer's disease, depression, anxiety syndrome, Parkinson's disease, and prion diseases, such as BSE, scrapie, and Creutzfeldt–Jakob disease.[6]

Figure 1 shows the correlation between glyphosate usage and rates of autism, tracking services received by autistic children under the Individuals with Disabilities Education Act (IDEA).[7]

The causes for the neurological disorders have been linked to glyphosate's impact on gut bacteria, metal chelation, and P450 inactivation.[8] Given the pervasive use of this chemical, it is fairly easy to come into contact with glyphosate in a number of ways: by direct absorption through the skin, by eating foods treated with it, or by drinking water contaminated with it. In one severe case, a fifty-four-year-old man who accidentally sprayed himself with glyphosate developed disseminated skin lesions six hours after the accident. One month later, he developed a symmetrical parkinsonian syndrome.[9] A 2015 review of the literature on glyphosate, indicated that the chemical, depending on dose and exposure time, affects the development of embryos, is capable of forming tumors and adversely affects the liver and kidneys.[10]

Glyphosate, Cancer, and the Microbiome

Because of the growing body of research on glyphosate, the World Health Organization International Agency for Research on

Cancer classified glyphosate as a probable carcinogen in humans.[11] Possible cancers linked to glyphosate exposure include non-Hodgkin lymphoma, renal tubule carcinoma, pancreatic islet-cell adenoma, and skin tumors.[12] A 2013 study of the effects of glyphosate on chickens found that exposure disrupted the ratio of good microbes to harmful microbes. As a result, there was an increase in pathogenic bacteria[13]. While the relationship between the microbiome of the intestine and overall human health is still unclear, current research suggests that disruption of the microbiome could cause diseases such as metabolic disorder, diabetes, depression, autism, cardiovascular disease, and autoimmune disease.[1]

Glyphosate and Chelation

Chelation is a process that binds ions and molecules to metal ions. Glyphosate acts as a chelating agent, particularly with calcium. As a result, glyphosate accumulates in bones, a fact admitted by Monsato.[14] Glyphosate has been found in the intestines, livers, muscles, spleens, and kidneys of slaughter animals. Additionally, chronically ill humans show significantly higher glyphosate residues in urine than healthy humans.[15] The chelating action of glyphosate with other metals appears to play a key role in an epidemic of kidney disease in Sri Lanka, India, and Central America.[16] These chelates may not be detected by common analytical chemistry methods that only detect free glyphosate, thus dramatically reducing estimates of glyphosate persistence in the environment when metals are high (for example, in clay soil or hard water).[1]

Testing for Glyphosate

Because glyphosate has been linked to many chronic health conditions, testing for glyphosate exposure and particularly the level of exposure is important. The Great Plains Laboratory is the only CLIA (Clinical Laboratory Improvement Amendments) certified lab currently performing a test for glyphosate in urine. This Glyphosate Test can be performed on a urine sample.

Other Problems with Glyphosate

In addition to the chelation ability of glyphosate, it inhibits the synthesis of tryptophan, phenylalanine, and tyrosine in plants, a primary source of these amino acids. Humans also require bacteria to maintain a healthy immune system. Glyphosate decreases the number of good bacteria, such as bifidobacterial and lactobacilli, in the gut, which allows for the overgrowth of harmful bacteria, such as campylobacter and C. difficile.[17]

The following case study is from The Great Plains Laboratory. A female patient suffering from depression did a Glyphosate Test and an Organic Acids Test (OAT). Her glyphosate result was 2.99, which was over the 95th percentile. The coincidence of depression and exposure to glyphosate has been confirmed with research.[5]

When glyphosate exposure reduces good bacteria, C. difficile that produces the toxin 4-cresol invades. The OAT measures this invasion. The toxin 4-cresol suppresses dopamine beta-dyroxylase Research has shown that 4-cresol inhibits dopamine beta-hydroxylase.[13] Dopamine beta-hydroxylase converts dopamine to norepinephrine. The OAT measures both homovanillic acid (dopamine metabolite) and vanillylmandelic acid (norepinephrine metabolite). The Great Plains Laboratory has observed that patients with a high 4-cresol value have elevated homovanillic acid, which indicates an inability to convert dopamine to norepinephrine, which may have been the cause of the patient's depression. The results from the aforementioned patient were consistent with these other results. The recommendations for this patient were to treat her glyphosate exposure and to treat her C. difficile infection.

The results from the Great Plains Laboratory tests are indicative of why using the Organic Acids Test and Glyphosate Test together is so valuable. Treatment of glyphosate toxicity should focus on determining the route of introduction and avoiding future exposure. Eating organic, non-GMO (genetically modified organism) foods and drinking reverse osmosis water are two of the best ways to avoid glyphosate. People who eat organic food have considerably lower concentrations of glyphosate in the urine.[8] Drinking extra water may also be beneficial since glyphosate is water soluble, but that water should be filtered to remove pesticides or, ideally, be treated by reverse osmosis or the Multipure[TM] solid carbon block technology with the 401 Emerging Compounds certification.

The use of glyphosate is so pervasive that it is virtually impossible to completely avoid exposure to it. More than 90% of corn and soy used are now of the GMO type. In addition, non-GMO wheat is commonly treated with glyphosate as a drying procedure. Glyphosate is somewhat volatile and a high percentage of rain samples also contained glyphosate.[8]

Summary

High correlations exist between glyphosate usage and numerous chronic illnesses, including autism. Other disease incidences with high correlations include hypertension, stroke, diabetes, obesity, lipoprotein metabolism disorder, Alzheimer's, senile dementia, Parkinson's, multiple sclerosis, inflammatory bowel disease, intestinal infections, end stage renal disease, acute kidney failure, cancers of the thyroid, liver, bladder, pancreas, kidney, and myeloid leukemia. Correlations are not causations, yet they raise concern over the use of a chemical to which all life on earth appears to be exposed. Testing for glyphosate along with specific markers in the Organic Acids Test can both help determine the level of exposure to glyphosate and guide you toward the most optimal treatment.

Treatment of glyphosate toxicity should focus on determining the route of introduction and avoiding future exposure. Eating non-GMO (genetically modified organism) foods and drinking reverse osmosis water or water going through a Multipure™ solid carbon filter are two of the best ways to avoid glyphosate. A recent study showed that people eating organic food had considerably lower concentrations of glyphosate in the urine.

Reference List

1. Shaw W, Pratt-Hyatt M. The importance of testing for glyphosate: the world's most widely used herbicide. *Toxic Chemicals* Jan 23, 2017. https://www.greatplainslaboratory.com/articles-1/2017/1/23/the-importance-of-testing-for-glyphosate-the-worlds-most-widely-used-herbicide. Accessed Feb 9, 2018.
2. Bradberry SM, Proudfoot AT, Vale JA. Glyphosate poisoning. *Toxicol Rev.* 2004;23(3):159-67.
3. U.S. Department of Veteran Affairs. *Agent orange.* June 2, 1017.

https://www.publichealth.va.gov/exposures/agentorange/.Ac
cessed Feb 9, 2018.

4. Mesnage R, Defarge N, Spiroux de Vendômois J, Sérlini GE. Major pesticides are more toxic to human cells than their declared active principles. *Biomed Res Int*. 2014, doi: 10.1155/2014/179691.

5. Samsel A, Seneff S. Glyphosate, pathways to modern diseases II: Celiac sprue and gluten intolerance. *Interdiscip Toxicol*. 2013; 6:159-184. doi: 10.2478/intox-2013-0026.

6. Samsel A, Seneff S. Glyphosate, pathways to modern diseases III: Manganese, neurological diseases, and associated pathologies. *Surg Neurol Int*. 2015; 6: 45. doi: 10.4103/2152-7806.153876.

7. Swanson NL, Leu A, Abrahamson J, and Wallet B. Genetically engineered crops, glyphosate and the deterioration of health in the United States of America. *Journal of Organic Systems*. 2014; 9(2):6-37. https://www.researchgate.net/publication/283462716_Ge netically_engineered_crops_glyphosate_and_the_deteriorati on_of_health_in_the_United_States_of_America. Accessed Feb 9, 2018.

8. Krüger M, Schledorn P, Schrödl W, Hoppe HW, Lutz W, Shehata AA. Detection of Glyphosate Residues in Animals and Humans. *J Environ Anal Toxicol*. 2014; 4:2. doi:10.4172/2161- 0525.1000210.

9. Barbosa ER, Leiros da Costa MD, Bacheschi LA, Scaff M, Leite CC. Parkinsonism after glycine-derivative exposure [ABSTRACT]. *Mov Disord* 2001; 16: 565-568. https://www.ncbi.nlm.nih.gov/pubmed/11391760. Accessed Feb 9, 2018.

10. Mesnage R, Defarge N, Spiroux de Vendômois J, Séralini GE. Potential toxic effects of glyphosate and its commercial formulations below regulatory limits. *Food Chem Toxicol* 2015 Oct; 84:133-53. doi: 10.1016/j.fct.2015.08.012.

11. Guyton KZ, Loomis D, Grosse Y et al. Carcinogenicity of tetrachlorvinphos, parathion, malathion, diazinon, and glyphosate. *Lancet Oncol* 2015 May;16(5):490-1. doi: 10.1016/S1470-2045(15)7014-8.

12. Williams M. Glyphosate as a cause of many chronic health problems. *Proposed Specific Regulatory Level Chemical Causing Cancer: Glyphosate.* June 10, 2017. https://oehha.ca.gov/proposition-65/comments/proposed-specific-regulatory-level-chemical-causing-cancer-glyphosate-265. Accessed Feb 9, 2018.
13. Shehata AA, Schrödl W, Aldin AA, Hafez HM, Krüger M. The effect of glyphosate on potential pathogens and beneficial members of poultry microbiota in vitro. *Curr Microbiol.* 2013 Apr;66(4):350-8. doi: 0.1007/s00284-012-0277-2.
14. Mcevoy M. Bone broth, collagen, and glyphosate toxicity. *Metabolic Healing: Empowering Your Health* Aug 21, 2017. https://metabolichealing.com/bone-broth-collagen-glyphosate-toxicity/. Accessed Feb 10, 2018.
15. Krüger M, Schledorn P, Schrödl W, Hoppe HW, Lutz W, Shahata A. A. Detection of glyphosate residues in animals and humans. *J Environ Anal Toxicol* 2014; 4:210. doi: 10.4172/2161-0525.1000210.
16. Jayasumana C, Gunatilake S, Senanayake P. Glyphosate, hard water and nephrotoxic metals: are they the culprits behind the epidemic of chronic kidney disease of unknown etiology in Sri Lanka? *Int. J. Environ. Res. Public Health* 2014; 11:2125-2147. doi:10.3390/ijerph110202125.
17. The Detox Project. *Glyphosate and Roundup negatively affect gut bacteria.* 2018. https://detoxproject.org/glyphosate/glyphosate-and-roundup-negatively-affect-gut-bacteria/. Accessed Feb 10, 2018.
18. DeWolf WE Jr. Inactivation of dopamine beta-hydroxylase by p-cresol: isolation and characterization of covalently modified active site peptides. *Biochemistry* 1988;27: 9093-9101. doi: 10.1021/bi00426a005.
19. Shaw W. Elevated urinary glyphosate and clostridia metabolites with altered dopamine metabolism in triplets with autism spectrum disorder or suspected seizure disorder: a case study. *Integr Med (Encinitas)* Feb 2017; 16(1): 50-57. https://www.ncbi.nlm.nih.gov/pubmed/28223908. Accessed Feb 13, 2018.

Chapter 10: Porphyrins

Porphyrins are generated as the body builds hemoglobin, the compound that carries oxygen in blood cells. Porphyrin (from the Greek word for purple) consists of four ring compounds joined together—a structure conducive to holding a metal ion in its center, iron in the heme porphyrin of hemoglobin, and magnesium in chlorophyll. Small amounts of several porphyrins appear in urine normally. Certain hereditary diseases and environmental or nutritional influences alter the relative amounts of each porphyrin. Acute, or hepatic, porphyria affects the nervous system, creating a host of symptoms including hallucinations, depression, anxiety, and paranoia.[1]

Porphyrins are proteins involved in the formation of heme measured in urine. Heme is essential for the proper function of many proteins including oxygen transport, energy production, and detoxification. Proper porphyrin production is essential for the body's capacity to detoxify toxins. Testing for porphyrins is a particularly good way to assess for heavy metal toxicity because their elevation indicates a toxic level of heavy metals.[2]

Symptoms of toxicity
- Fatigue/weakness
- Chemical sensitivity
- Irritability
- Anxiety
- Memory loss
- Insomnia
- Numbness and tingling in hands and feet
- Tremors
- Gastrointestinal issues
- Loss of appetite

Sources of toxicants
- Fish
- Amalgams
- Polluted air and soil
- Fluorescent bulbs
- Paints
- Pottery

- Ground water
- Tobacco
- Vaccinations

The Porphyrins Profile

The Porphyrins Profile is a urine test that helps to identify the severity of heavy metal toxicity or organic chemical exposure in patients. This test is available through Genova Diagnostics and Great Plains Laboratory through the GPL-Tox: Toxic Non-metal Chemical Profile. Chemical exposure and a heavy toxic burden can have physiological effects that result in impaired metabolism and cellular function.

Porphyrin testing helps identify the following.
- Levels of biochemical damage caused by toxicant exposure
- Physiologic burden of a person's level of toxins
- Levels of porphyrin elevation correlated with levels of toxic interference
- Toxicity of patients before and during chelation therapy
- Toxicity of therapeutic drugs

This testing is particularly important for someone who has been diagnosed with autism spectrum, given the role of mercury in that spectrum.[3]

Reference List

1. World Heritage Encyclopedia. Hereditary erythropoietic porphyria. *Newspapers Library*. 2018. http://newspaperslibrary.org/articles/eng/Hereditary_erythropoietic_porphyria. Accessed Feb 13, 2018.

2. Shaw W. *Porphyrin testing and heavy metal toxicity; unresolved questions and concerns.* doi: 10.1.1.590.825&rep=rep1&type=pdf.

3. Kem JK, Geier D A, Sykes LK, Haley BE, Geier MR. The relationship between mercury and autism: a comprehensive review and discussion. *Journal of Trace Elements in Medicine and Biology* Sep 2016; 37: 8-24. https://www.sciencedirect.com/science/article/pii/S0946672X16300931. Accessed Feb 13, 2018.

Chapter 11: GPL-MycoTox Profile

Mycotoxins, metabolites produced by fungi-like mold that can infest buildings, vehicles, and foods, are some of the most prevalent toxins in the environment. In the European Union, 20% of all grains harvested have been found to be contaminated with mycotoxins. Most human exposure comes through food ingestion or airborne exposure. Fungi are able to grow on almost any surface, especially if the environment is warm and wet. Inner wall materials of buildings, wall paper, fiber glass insulation, ceiling tiles, and gypsum support are all good surfaces for fungi to colonize. Mold can also grow on wallpaper, carpet, fabric, and upholstery. Mold grows well on organic products, such as paper, wood, cardboard, and ceiling tiles. Unfortunately, mycotoxins are resistant to heat and many food processing procedures.

These fungi then release mycotoxins into the environment, causing symptoms of many different chronic diseases. Diseases and symptoms linked to mycotoxin exposure include fever, pneumonia-like symptoms, heart disease, rheumatic disease, asthma, sinusitis, cancer, memory loss, vision loss, chronic fatigue, skin rashes, depression, ADHD, anxiety, and liver damage.[1]

Species of Mold Tested by GPL-MycoTox

Aspergillus
Aspergillus, the most prevalent mold group in the environment, causes billions of dollars of in damage to crops and livestock. Two of the most common *Aspergillus* mycotoxins are aflatoxin and ochratoxin. The main target of these toxins is the liver. These toxins have been found in all major cereal crops including peanuts, corn, cotton, millet, rice, sorghum, sunflower seeds, wheat, and a variety of spices. They are also found in eggs, milk, and meat from animals fed contaminated grains. Diseases caused by *Aspergillus* are called aspergillosis. The most common route of infection is through the respiratory system. *Aspergillus* can cause severe asthma when the mold colonizes the lung, forming a granulomatous disease.[2,3]

Penicillum

With over 200 species of *penicillium*, it is the most common fungi found in soil. While some varieties are toxic, others are beneficial, such as those found in ripened cheeses like Brie and Stilton and the drug penicillin, *penicillium chrysogenum,* which also occurs in most household molds. In the home, penicillium can be found in wallpaper, carpet, furniture, and fiberglass insulation and may grow on different foods, particularly citrus. Because it thrives in low humidity, it is a common mold. It produces the common mycotoxin ochratoxin (OTA), nephrotoxic that damages the kidneys and is also carcinogenic.[4,5]

Stachybotrys

Stachybotrys, a greenish-black mold, grows on materials with high cellulose and low nitrogen content like gypsum board, paper, fiberboard, and ceiling tiles. *Stachybotrys* produces the highly toxic macrocyclic trichothecene mycotoxins. Two of the more common mycotoxins produced by *Stachybotrys* are roridin E and verrucarin. Additional mycotoxins include nine phenylspirodrimanes and cyclosporine, which are potent immunosuppressors.[6]

Fusarium

Fusarium fungi causes a broad spectrum of infections in humans. Exposure to mycotoxins from *Fusarium* can lead to both acute and chronic effects. Because it requires lower temperatures for growth than *Aspergillus,* it grows best in temperate climates. Humans may encounter it from its growth on different grains. *Fusarium's* major mycotoxins are zearalenone (ZEN) and fumonisin. ZEN possesses estrogenic effects and has been implicated in reproductive disorders.[7]

Toxins produced by mold/fungus

Aflatoxin M1 (AFM1)

Aflatoxin M1 (AFM1) is the main metabolite of aflatoxin B1, which is a mycotoxin produced by the mold species Aspergillus in grains. AFM1 is found in milk and milk products.[8,10] Aflatoxins are some of the most carcinogenic substances in the environment. In cases of lung aspergilloma, aflatoxin has been found in human tissue specimens.[9] Aflatoxin poisoning can cause nausea, vomiting, and abdominal pain, convulsions, cerebral edema, blood abnormalities, liver damage and cancer in some animals,[10] damage to the kidneys and heart, and death.[11] Aflatoxin has been shown to inhibit leucocyte proliferation. Aflatoxicosis is primarily a problem in developing nations. Since its symptoms are very much like those of virus, the condition may be misdiagnosed.[11] The toxicity of Aflatoxin is increased in the presence of ochratoxin and zearalenone. Aflatoxin susceptibility is dependent on multiple different factors such as age, sex, and diet.

Enniatin B1

Enniatin B1 is a fungal metabolite categorized as cyclohexa depsipeptides toxin produced by the fungus Fusarium, which is a common cereal contaminant. Enniatin B1 may have potential as a treatment of cancer.[12] There are limited studies on any toxic effects.

Ochratoxin A (OTA)

Ochratoxin A (OTA) is a nephrotoxic, immunotoxic, and carcinogenic mycotoxin, produced by Aspergillus and Penicillium species. While OTA causes nephrotoxicity and renal tumors in some animal species, its effects on human health are less well-defined. OTA may lead to kidney disease and adverse neurological effects. Dopamine levels in the brain of mice have been shown to be decreased after exposure to OTA. It is a naturally occurring foodborne mycotoxin because of poor storage or drying. Primary contamination comes from ingestion of contaminated foods: cereals, grape juices, dairy, spices, wine, dried vine fruit, and coffee.[13] Exposure to OTA can also come from inhalation exposure in water-damaged buildings.

Rordidin E

Roridin E, produced by the soil fungus *Myrothecium uerucaria,* may be implicated in animal and human infections via contaminated food. Adverse effects have been recorded in the kidney and livers of rats.[14]

Sterignatocystin (STG)

A 2018 report by the Joint FAO/WHO Expert Committee on Food Additives concluded that Sterigmatocystin (STG) is genotoxic and carcinogenic.[15] It is produced by several species of mold, including Aspergillus, Penicillium, and Bipolaris. STG has been found in the dust from damp carpets. It has been found in samples of a variety of foods, including pistachios, pecans, wheat, cheese, spices, green coffee beans, soybeans, and processed foods containing grains, such as bread and animal feed.[16] Its toxic effects are similar to those of aflatoxin B1. In test animals, chronic symptoms include hepatomas (cancer of cells in the liver), pulmonary tumors, renal lesions, and alterations in the liver and kidneys. No definite links have been established between STG and cancer in humans.[16] However, oxidative stress becomes measurably elevated during STG exposure, which causes a depletion of antioxidants such as glutathione, particularly in the liver.

Trichothecene

Trichothecene, produced by the mold species Fusarium, Myrothecium, and Stachybotrys (i.e. black mold), is frequently found in buildings with water damage but can also be found in contaminated corn, barley, sunflower seeds, rye, and wheat. Animals exposed to elevated doses of this mycotoxin experience nausea, vomiting, and diarrhea. Prolonged exposure causes reduced growth and damage to internal organs—spleen, thymus, liver, and heart.[18] One form is a very toxic compound that inhibits protein biosynthesis by preventing peptidyl transferase activity.[19] Trichothecene mycotoxins been used as biological warfare agents and the effects resemble radiation exposure. Even low levels of exposure to macrocyclic trichothecenes can cause severe neurological damage, immunosuppression, endocrine disruption, cardiovascular problems, and gastrointestinal distress.[20]

Verrucarin A

Verrucarin A (VRA), a macrocyclic trichothecene mycotoxin produced from Stachybotrys, Fusarium, and Myrothecium, is produced on grains like wheat, oats or maize, but some molds producing this mycotoxin can grow in buildings, contributing to the health problems of occupants.[21] VRA is a small, amphipathic molecule that can move passively across cell membranes, causing inflammation. The primary tissues affected by VRA are intestinal and gastric mucosa, bone marrow, and spleen. VRA causes damage to human cells by inhibiting protein and DNA synthesis, disrupting mitochondrial functions, and by producing oxidative stress (due to generation of free radicals). Exposure to VRA can cause immunological problems, vomiting, skin dermatitis, and hemorrhagic lesions.[22]

Zearalenone (ZEA)

Zearalenone (ZEA) is a mycotoxin produced by the mold species Fusarium that grows primarily on wheat and maize. Animal studies show that ZEA has estrogenic activity higher than other non-steroid isoflavones like soy and clover and exposure to ZEA can lead to reproductive changes. There is also additional bilirubin concentration in the blood, indicating some liver toxicity.[23] ZEA, like estrogen and other endocrine disruptors, is an immunotoxic compound. In human case studies, chronic exposure to ZEA resulted in early onset of puberty in girls.[24]

ADVANTAGES OF THE GPL-MYCOTOX PROFILE
- GPL-MycoTOX screens for seven different mycotoxins, from four species of mold, in one urine sample.
- GPL-MycoTOX is the most comprehensive and competitively priced mycotoxin test available.
- GPL-MycoTOX uses the power of advanced mass spectrometry (MS/MS), which is necessary to detect lower levels of these fungal toxins. This test is optimal for follow up testing to ensure that detoxification therapies have been successful.
- GPL-MycoTOX pairs perfectly with the Organic Acids Test (OAT), GPL-TOX (Toxic Non-Metal Chemical Profile), Phospholipase A2 Activity Test, and the Glyphosate Test. This gives you comprehensive testing to assess exposure to common environmental toxins and the damage that can be caused by this exposure, all at a great value, and all from one urine sample.[25]

Recommendations for Treatment

I provide my patients test kits to take to their homes and offices to check for mold growth. If any is present, I recommend testing. Approximately 75-80% of my patients in the Tampa Bay

---

85

area come back with mold growing in the petri dishes. If mold is present, I use the GPL-MycoTox Profiles. These are the recommendations I make for moderate to high levels of mycotoxins to help the body eliminate the toxins and prevent future exposures.

Step 1: Eliminate or reduce exposure to mold. The majority of exposures result from contaminated food, skin contact, and inhalation of spore-borne toxins that is often caused by water-damaged buildings. Inhalation of spore-borne toxins can be limited by detecting and eliminating damp and moldy environments, both indoor and outdoor. As mentioned previously, mold spores can enter homes through open windows, vents, doorways, and heating and air conditioning systems. Mold can be controlled by cleaning and drying after water intrusion; having proper ventilation for showers, laundry, and cooking areas; making sure that windows, roofs, and pipes are free of leaks; and by controlling humidity levels. After moisture problems have been alleviated, I recommend that mold removal be performed by a licensed contractor because attempts to remove mold may cause mold spores to scatter and spread. Also, treating mold without proper ventilation may result in health problems caused by the release of mycotoxins from the mold spores.

Step 2: Include an ActivePure™ air purification system in the home and work place.

Step 3: Provide fluid support to prevent dehydration.

Step 4: Instigate of carrots, parsnips, celery, and parsley to reduce the carcinogenic effects of mold.

Step 5: Reduce the absorption of mold found in food by taking bentonite clay and zeolite clay.

Step 6: Supplement with chlorophyllin, zinc, A, E, C, NAC, rosmarinic acid, and liposomal reduced glutathione alone or in combination to mitigate the oxidative effects of mold.

I have a combination of specific products I recommend for patients experiencing problems with mold.

Reference List

1. Brewer JH, Thrasher JH, Hooper D. Chronic illness associated with mold and mycotoxins: is naso-sinus fungal biofilm the culprit? *Toxins (Basel)* 2014 Jan; 6(1): 66-80.

2. The Aspergillus Website. https://www.aspergillus.org.uk/. Accessed 2 April 2018.

3. Pratt-Hyatt M. Mycotoxins: the hidden threat of mold to our bodies and brains. *The Townsend Newsletter: The Examiner of Alternative Medicine,* Oct 2017. http://www.townsendletter.com/Oct2017/mycotoxin1017.html. Accessed Apr 2, 2018.

4. *Penicillium.* http://website.nbm-mnb.ca/mycologywebpages/Moulds/Penicillium.html. Accessed Apr 2, 2018.

5. Kung'u J. *Penicillium species as indoor contaminants.* http://www.moldbacteriaconsulting.com/fungi/penicillium-species-as-indoor-air.html. Accessed Apr 2, 2018.

6. Nelson BD. *Stachybotrys chartarum*: the toxic indoor mold. *The Phytopathological Society,* Feb 1999. http://www.apsnet.org/publications/apsnetfeatures/Pages/Stachybotrys.aspx. Accessed Apr 2, 2018.

7. Nucci M, Annaissie E. *Fusarium* infections in immunocompromised patients. *Clinic Microbio Rev* 2007 Oct; 20(4): 695-704. doi: 10.1128/CMR.00014-07.

8. National Center for Biotechnology. Aflotoxin m1. *Open Chemistry Database.* https://pubchem.ncbi.nlm.nih.gov/compound/aflatoxin_m1#section=Top. Accessed Apr 3, 2018.

9. Kosmidis C, Denning DW. *Aspergilloma.* https://www.aspergillus.org.uk/content/aspergilloma-0. Accessed Apr 4, 2018.

10. U.S. Food and Drug Administration. *CPG Sec. 527.400 whole milk, lowfat milk, skim milk—Aflatoxin M1.* https://www.fda.gov/ICECI/ComplianceManuals/CompliancePolicyGuidanceManual/ucm074482.htm. Accessed Apr 4, 2018.

11. Cheprosov A. Aflatoxin poisoning: symptoms, treatments, and effects. Chapter 4. *Study.com.*

https://study.com/academy/lesson/aflatoxin-poisoning-symptoms-treatment-effects.html. Accessed Apr 4, 2018.

12. Feudijo FT, Dometshuber R, Lemmens N, Hoffman O, Lemmens-Gruber R, Berger W. Beauvericin and enniatin: emerging toxins or remedies?. *World Mycotoxin Journal* 2010 Nov 4; 3(4): 415-430. doi: 10.3920/WMJ2010.1245.

13. Bui-Kimke TR, Wu F. Ochatroxin A and human health risk: a review of the evidence. *Crit Rev Food Sci Nutr* 2015 Nov 10; 55(13): 1860-1869. doi: 10.1080/10408398.2012.724480.

14. Chrevatidis A. Mycotoxins/occurrence and determination. *Encyclopedia of Food Sciences and Nutrition, 2nd ed,* 2003: 4089-4096. doi: 10.1016/B0-12-227055-X/00822-1.

15. World Health Organization. Sterigmatocystin. *Evaluations of the Joint FAO/WHO expert committee on food additives.* http://apps.who.int/food-additives-contaminants-jecfa-database/chemical.aspx?chemID=6458. Accessed Apr 4, 2018.

16. Sterigmatocystin. *Toxic Black Mould.* http://www.blackmould.me.uk/sterigmatocystin.html. Accessed Apr 4, 2018.

17. Omar HEDM, Sawi NME, Meki AR. Acute toxicity of the mycotoxin roridin E on liver and kidney of rats. *J Appl Anim Res* 1997; 12: 143-152. https://www.tandfonline.com/doi/pdf/10.1080/09712119.1997.9706200. Accessed Apr 4, 2018.

18. Mbundi L, Gallar-Ayala H, Khan MR, Barber JL, Losada S, Busquets R. Advances in the analysis of challenging food contaminants. *Advances in Molecular Toxicology* 2014. doi.org/10.1016/B978-0-444-63406-1.00002-7.

19. McCormick SP, Stanley AM, Stover NA, Alexander NJ. Trichothecenes: from simple to complex mycotoxins. *Toxins (Basel)* 2011 Jul; 3(7): 802-814. doi: 10.3390/toxins3070802.

20. Hashek WM, Beasely VR. Trichothecene mycotoxins. In Ramesh C. Gupta, ed. *Handbook of Toxicology of Warfare Agents.* Amsterdam: Elsevier, 2009: 353-369.

21. Genome Canada. *Verrucarin A (T3D3720).* http://www.t3db.ca/toxins/T3D3720. Accessed Apr 9, 2018.

22. Kankkuken P, Rintahaka J, Aalto A. et. al. Trichothechene mycotoxins activate inflammatory response in human macrophages. The Journal of Immunology, 2009, 182: 6418–6425. http://www.jimmunol.org/content/jimmunol/182/10/6418.full .pdf. Accessed Apr 9, 2018.

23. Denli M, Blandon JC, Salado S, Guynot ME, Perez JF. Effect of dietary zearalenone on the performance, reproduction tract and serum biochemistry in young rats. *Open Source.* Oct 18, 2016. https://www.tandfonline.com/doi/pdf/10.1080/09712119.201 6.1251929https://www.tandfonline.com/doi/pdf/10.1080/097 12119.2016.1251929. Accessed Apr 9, 2018.

24. Hueza IM, Raspantini PCF, Raspantini LER, Latorre AO, Górniak SL. Zearalenone, an estrogen mycotoxin, is an immunotoxic compound. *Toxins (Basel)* 2014 Mar; 6(3): 1080-1095. doi: 10.3390/toxins6031080.

25. GPL-MycoTOX Profile. The Great Plains Laboratory, Inc. https://www.greatplainslaboratory.com/gplmycotox. Accessed Apr 9, 2018.

Chapter 12: GPL-TOX: Toxic Non-Metal Chemical Profile

As I have discussed in my previous publications, each of us are exposed to hundreds of toxic chemicals daily through products like pharmaceuticals, pesticides, packaged foods, household products, and environmental pollution. This exposure to chemical-laden products and toxic food, air, and water pollutants has accelerated rates of chronic illnesses like cancer, heart disease, chronic fatigue syndrome, chemical sensitivity, autism spectrum disorders, ADD/AD(H)D, autoimmune disorders, Parkinson's disease, and Alzheimer's disease.

Nonmetal Toxins and Metabolites

Phthalates are perhaps the most widespread group of toxic environmental chemicals. They are commonly found in aftershave lotions, aspirin, cosmetics, detergents, foods microwaved with plastic covers, oral pharmaceutical drugs, intravenous products prepared in plastic bags, hair sprays, insecticides, insect repellents, nail polish, nail polish remover, skin care products, adhesives, explosives, lacquer, janitorial products, perfumes, paper coatings, printing inks, safety glass, and varnishes. Phthalates have been implicated in reproductive damage, depressed leukocyte function, and cancer. Phthalates have also been found to impede blood coagulation, lower testosterone, and alter sexual development in children. Low levels of phthalates can feminize the male brain of the fetus, while high levels can hyper-masculinize the developing male brain. (See Chapter 7 on Phthalates.) *Monoethyl Phthalate (MEP)* from diethyl phthalate is the most abundant phthalate metabolite found in urine. Diethyl phthalate is used in plastic products. Elevated values indicate exposure from various possible sources. Elimination of phthalates may be accelerated by sauna treatment.

Vinyl Chloride is an intermediate in the synthesis of several commercial chemicals, including polyvinyl chloride (PVC). Exposure to vinyl chloride may cause central nervous system depression, nausea, headache, dizziness, liver damage, degenerative bone changes, thrombocytopenia, enlargement of the spleen, and death.

Benzene, a widespread environmental organic solvent, is a by-product of all sources of combustion, including cigarette smoke and numerous industrial processes. It is released as a vapor from synthetic materials. Extremely toxic, it is mutagenic and carcinogenic. High exposures to benzene cause symptoms of nausea, vomiting, dizziness, lack of coordination, central nervous system depression, and death. It can also cause hematological abnormalities. *N-acetyl phenyl cysteine (NAP)* is a metabolite of benzene. Treatment consists of removing sources of exposure.

Pyrethrins are widely used insecticides. Exposure during pregnancy doubles the likelihood of autism. They may affect neurological development, disrupt hormones, induce cancer, and suppress the immune system. *3-Phenoxybenzoic Acid (3PBA)* is a metabolite of pyrethroid insecticides. Elimination can be accelerated by sauna treatment.

Xylenes (dimethylbenzenes)—solvents found not only in common products such as paints, lacquers, pesticides, cleaning fluids, fuel and exhaust fumes, but also in perfumes and insect repellents—are oxidized in the liver and bound to glycine before eliminated in urine. High xylene levels may be due to the use of certain perfumes and insect repellents. High exposures to xylene create an increase in oxidative stress, causing symptoms such as nausea, vomiting, dizziness, central nervous system depression, and death. Occupational exposure is often found in pathology laboratories where xylene is used for tissue processing. Exposure to xylenes generates methylhippuric acid isomers--*2-Methylhippuric Acid (2MHA), 3-Methylhippuric Acid (3MHA), 4-Methylhippuric Acid (4MHA)*. Avoid/reduce exposure to these substances.

Styrene, used in the manufacturing of plastics and building materials, is found in car exhaust fumes. Polystyrene and its copolymers are commonly used as food-packaging materials. The ability of styrene monomer to leach from polystyrene packaging to food has been reported. Occupational exposure due to inhalation of large amounts of styrene adversely impacts the central nervous system, causes concentration problems, muscle weakness, tiredness and nausea, and irritates the mucous membranes of the eyes, nose, and throat. *Phenylglyoxylic Acid (PGO)* is the result of exposure to environmental styrene. Reduce exposure by eliminating use of plastics and Styrofoam containers for cooking, reheating, eating, or drinking. Supplement with glutathione and N-acetyl cysteine (NAC) to accelerate elimination.

Organophosphates, one of the most toxic groups of substances, are often used as biochemical weapons and terrorist agents as well as in pesticides. They are inhibitors of cholinesterase enzymes that lead to overstimulation and abnormal behavior, including aggression and depression. Children exposed to these chemicals have more than twice the risk of developing pervasive developmental disorder (PDD) and autism spectrum disorder. Maternal organophosphate exposure has been associated with various adverse outcomes including having shorter pregnancies and children with impaired reflexes. *Diphenyl Phosphate*, a metabolite of the organophosphate flame retardant triphenyl phosphate (TPHP), is used in plastics, electronic equipment, nail polish, and resins. TPHP can cause endocrine disruption. Studies have also linked it to reproductive and developmental problems. *Dimethylphosphate (DMP) & Diethylphosphate (DEP)* are major metabolites of many organophosphate pesticides. Reduce exposure by eating organic foods and avoiding use of pesticides in your home or garden. Living near agricultural areas or golf courses and areas regularly sprayed with pesticides increases exposure. Elimination of organophosphates can be accelerated by sauna treatment.

MTBE (and ETBE), a gasoline additive used to improve octane ratings, has been demonstrated to cause hepatic, kidney, and central nervous system toxicity, peripheral neurotoxicity, and cancer in animals. Exposure to these compounds is most likely due to groundwater contamination, inhalation, or skin exposure to gasoline or its vapors and exhaust fumes. ETBE is guilty by association with MTBE because of its similar chemical formula. *2-Hydroxyisobutyric Acid (2HIB)* is the major metabolite of gasoline octane enhancers, such as MTBE and ETBE. Elevated levels indicate environmental exposure and very high values have been reported in genetic disorders.

2, 4-Dicholorophenoxyacetic (2,4-D), a very common herbicide that was part of Agent Orange used by the U.S. for defoliation during the Vietnam War, is today most commonly used in agriculture on genetically modified foods and as a weed killer for lawns. Exposure to 2, 4-D via skin or oral ingestion is associated with neuritis, weakness, nausea, abdominal pain, headache, dizziness, peripheral neuropathy, stupor, seizures, brain damage, and impaired reflexes. It is also a known endocrine disruptor that can block hormone distribution and cause glandular breakdown. *2,4-Dichlorophenoxyacetic Acid (2,4-D)* is a metabolite. Reduce exposure by eating organic foods and avoiding use of pesticides in your home or garden.

Acrylamide can change or combine to form polyacrylamide, which is used in many industrial processes such as plastics, food packaging, cosmetics, nail polish, dyes, and treatment of drinking water. Food and cigarette smoke are also two major sources of exposure. Acrylamide has been found in foods like potato chips, French fries, and many others such as asparagus, potatoes, legumes, nuts, seeds, beef, eggs, and fish. Asparagine, which is found in these same foods, can produce acrylamide when cooked at high temperature in the presence of sugars. High levels of acrylamide can elevate a patient's risk of cancer. In addition, acrylamide is known to cause neurological damage. *N-acetyl-S-(2-carbamoylethyl)-cysteine* is a metabolite of acrylamide.. Supplementation with glutathione can assist in the elimination of this compound.

Perchlorate, used in the production of rocket fuel, missiles, fireworks, flares, explosives, fertilizers, and bleach, has been found in some water supplies and contaminates many food sources. It can disrupt the thyroid's ability to produce hormones. The EPA has also labeled perchlorate a likely human carcinogen. Patients who test high for perchlorate exposure can use a reverse osmosis water treatment system to remove the chemical from their water supply.

1,3 Butadiene, a chemical made from the processing of petroleum, is often a colorless gas with a mild gasoline-like odor. Most of it is used in the production of synthetic rubber. It is a known carcinogen and has been linked to increased risk of cardiovascular disease.

Individuals who come into contact with rubber, such as car tires, can absorb 1,3 Butadiene through the skin. The increased use of old tires in the production of crumb rubber playgrounds and athletic fields is quite troubling because children and athletes may be exposed to toxic chemicals this way. *N-Acetyl (3,4-Dihydroxybutyl) Cysteine (NABD)* is a metabolite of 1,3 butadiene.

Propylene Oxide—used in the production of plastics and as a fumigant, to make polyester resins for textile and construction industries, and in the preparation of lubricants, surfactants, and oil demulsifiers—has also been used as a food additive, an herbicide, a microbicide, an insecticide, a fungicide, and a miticide. Propylene oxide is a probable human carcinogen. *N-Acetyl (2,Hydroxypropl) Cysteine (NAHP)* is a metabolite of propylene oxide.

1-Bromopropane (1-BP), an organic solvent used for metal cleaning, foam gluing, and dry cleaning, is a neurotoxin as well as a reproductive toxin. Research indicates that exposure to 1-BP can cause sensory and motor deficits. Chronic exposure can lead to decreased cognitive function and impaired central nervous system. Acute exposure can lead to headaches. *N-Acetyl (Propyl) Cysteine (NAPR)* is a metabolite of 1-bromopropane.

Ethylene Oxide, used in agrochemicals detergents, pharmaceuticals, personal care products, and a sterilizing agent on rubber, plastics, and electronics, has been reported as a carcinogen. Chronic exposure to it is mutagenic to humans. People exposed to ethylene oxide show an increased incidence of breast cancer and leukemia. Caution is needed with ethylene oxide because it is an odorless at toxic levels. *2-Hydroxyethyl Mercapturic Acid (HEMA)* is a metabolite of ethylene oxide. Supplementation with glutathione should assist in the detoxification process of these chemicals.

Acrylonitrile, a colorless liquid with a pungent odor, is used in the production of acrylic fibers, resins, and rubber. Use of any of these products can lead to exposure to acrylonitrile. Smoking tobacco and cigarettes is another potential exposure. Exposure to acrylonitrile can lead to headaches, nausea, dizziness, fatigue, and chest pains. The European Union has classified acrylonitrile as a

---

carcinogen. *N-Acetyl (2-Cyanoethyl) Cysteine (NACE)* is a metabolite of acrylonitrile. Supplementation with glutathione should assist in the detoxification of acrylonitrile.

Tiglylglycine (TG) is a marker for mitochondrial dysfunction. Mutations of mitochondria DNA may result from exposure to toxic chemicals, infections, inflammation, and nutritional deficiencies. These mutations can result from exposure to toxic chemicals, infections, inflammation, and nutritional deficiencies. Mitochondria are important in all cells in the body but are especially important to organs that utilize large amounts of energy, such as the muscles, heart, and brain. The mitochondria also have several other important functions in the cell, including steroid synthesis, calcium regulation, free radical production, and the induction of apoptosis or programmed cell death, all of which are involved in the pathogenesis of numerous disorders. Disorders associated with mitochondrial dysfunction include autism, Parkinson's disease, and cancer.

GPL-TOX
Because exposure to environmental pollutants has been linked to many chronic diseases, The Great Plains Laboratory has created GPL-TOX, a toxic non-metal chemical profile that screens for the presence of 172 different toxic chemicals, including organophosphate pesticides, phthalates, benzene, xylene, vinyl chloride, pyrethroid insecticides, acrylamide, perchlorate, diphenyl phosphate, ethylene oxide, acrylonitrile, and more (see above list). This is one of the common panels I run to evaluate the body burden of environmental toxins. This profile also includes Tiglylglycine (TG), a marker for mitochondrial disorders resulting from mutations of mitochondrial DNA. These mutations can be caused by exposure to toxic chemicals, infections, inflammation, and nutritional deficiencies.
There are many advantages to using the GPL-TOX profile.
- GPL-TOX screens for 172 different environmental pollutants using 18 different metabolites from a single urine sample.
- GPL-TOX uses the power of advanced mass spectrometry (MS/MS), which is necessary to detect lower levels of certain genetic, mitochondrial, and toxic

chemical markers that conventional mass spectrometry often misses.

- GPL-TOX also includes Tiglylglycine, a marker for mitochondrial damage, which is often seen in chronic toxic chemical exposure.
- GPL-TOX pairs perfectly with the Organic Acids Test (OAT) and Glyphosate Test in the Enviro-TOX Panel. This panel offers comprehensive testing to assess exposure to common environmental toxins and the damage that can be caused by this exposure from one urine sample.

This is a list of conditions in alphabetic order for which I recommend the GPL-TOX panel.

- Alzheimer's Disease
- Amyotrophic Lateral Sclerosis (ALS)
- Anorexia Nervosa
- Anxiety Disorder
- Apraxia
- Arthritis
- Asthma
- Attention deficit (ADD)
- Attention deficit with hyperactivity (ADHD)
- Autism
- Autoimmune disorders
- Bipolar disorder
- Cancer
- Cerebral palsy
- Chronic fatigue syndrome
- Crohn's disease
- Depression
- Developmental disorder
- Down Syndrome
- Epilepsy
- Failure to thrive
- Fibromyalgia
- Genetic diseases
- Irritable bowel syndrome

- Learning disability
- Mitochondria disorder
- Multiple sclerosis
- Obsessive compulsive disorder (OCD)
- Occupational exposures
- Parkinson's disease
- Peripheral neuropathy
- Schizophrenia
- Seizure disorders
- Systemic lupus erythematosus
- Tic disorders
- Tourette syndrome
- Ulcerative colitis

There are several common considerations for positive findings in the GPL-TOX panel. If you have had a GPL-TOX profile and/or a Glyphosate test run and found moderate-high levels of any compounds, there are actions you can take to help your body eliminate the toxins and to prevent future exposures. The first steps to reducing the amount of toxins presently in the body are to switch to eating only organic food and drinking water that has common toxins, including pesticides filtered out.

Because most conventional food crops are exposed to larger and larger doses of pesticides and herbicides, you prevent exposure to hundreds of these toxicants by switching to organic. Many of these chemicals have also contaminated water supplies. To eliminate these contaminants, install a high-quality reverse osmosis water filtration system or solid carbon filter such as Multipure™. (See Chapter 14: Water Pollution Solutions).

The next step to avoiding future exposures is to change the products you use on a daily basis from food and beverage containers to beauty and cleaning products. Instead of using plastic water bottles and food containers, switch to glass or metal. Never microwave food in plastic or Styrofoam containers and do not drink hot beverages from plastic or Styrofoam cups. Make sure your shampoo, soaps, lotions, and other beauty products are free of phthalates. Use cleaning products made from natural green ingredients or make your own at home.

To eliminate toxins from the body, I highly recommend exercise and the use of saunas, especially infrared sauna therapy to rid many chemicals through sweat. Infrared sauna is superior to conventional sauna because it reaches deeper into the body, increasing the circulation in the blood vessels and causing the body to start to release many of the chemicals stored in body fat. The two supplements that are particularly useful in helping the body detoxify are glutathione, or its precursor N-acetyl cysteine, and Vitamin B3 (Niacin). Glutathione is one of the most common molecules used by the body to eliminate toxic chemicals. If you are constantly exposed to toxicants, your stores of glutathione could be depleted. The second supplement, Vitamin B3 (niacin), causes flushing from the blood vessels dilating, which is useful in the detoxification process. If sensitive to the flushing, start with the lowest recommended dose and work up from there.

For more information on detoxification, refer to the Conclusion at the end of the book.

Chapter 13: Symptoms/Conditions and Potential Causes

This chapter summarizes common signs and symptoms of poor health, cross references potential environmental causes, and directs you to the appropriate testing. The fact of the matter is that environmental toxins are having adverse effects on the majority of the population in the United States in varying degrees. Sadly, most people and their doctors are not aware of how severe this potential health threat is. Hopefully, this book, and others written in the same vein, will increase awareness. Because you are now one of the informed, you have the ability to investigate, make changes where needed, and take charge of your health for the better. It is my hope and desire that you use this information to protect you, your family, and other loved ones.

Substantially eliminating and reducing environmental toxins is essential for giving you a better chance at optimal health. Environmental toxins lead to nutritional deficiencies as the micronutrients needed to bind with and negate the toxin are used up at a faster rate than it is being replaced unless an individual knows what s/he need more of. Detoxification, anti-oxidation, and immune systems become overwhelmed. As a result, health problems develop, persist, and worsen. Three problems that occur while this is happening include compromise in the tight junctions in the small intestine leading to hyperpermability (leaky gut), compromise of the glycocalyx that protects the endothelial layer in the blood vessels, and a decrease in hormone levels. (See *13 Secrets to Optimal Aging.*)

My experience indicates that almost 80 % of the adult population in the U.S. has decreased thyroid function as documented by the thyroflex, an FDA cleared device that measures intracellular levels of T3 with a 98.5 % accuracy. Numerous environmental toxins, including mercury, arsenic, bromine, fluoride, perchlorates, BPAs, and phthalates, adversely affect the thyroid.

Environmental toxins can cause the following symptoms and conditions.

- Alzheimer's Disease
- Amyotrophic Lateral Sclerosis (ALS)
- Anorexia Nervosa
- Anxiety Disorder
- Apraxia

- Arthritis
- Asthma
- Attention deficit (ADD)
- Attention deficit with hyperactivity (ADHD)
- Autism
- Autoimmune disorders
- Behavioral disorders
- Bipolar disorder
- Cancer
- Cerebral palsy
- Chronic fatigue syndrome
- Chronic inflammation
- Crohn's disease
- Depression
- Developmental disorder
- Down Syndrome
- Epilepsy
- Failure to thrive
- Fibromyalgia
- Genetic diseases
- Hypothyroidism
- Hypertension
- Irritable bowel syndrome
- Learning disability
- Mitochondria disorder
- Multiple sclerosis
- Obsessive compulsive disorder (OCD)
- Occupational exposures
- Parkinson's disease
- Peripheral neuropathy
- Schizophrenia
- Seizure disorders
- Systemic lupus erythematosus
- Tic disorders
- Tourette syndrome
- Ulcerative colitis

If you have a chronic health problem, you should consider environmental testing as part of the process to differentiate the causes. The best strategy is threefold.

1. Identify environmental toxins.
2. Develop a plan to eliminate and/or reduce continued exposure.
3. Give your body the foods and nutrients it needs to detoxify it.

Chapter 14: NSF

NSF International is a not-for-profit corporation founded in 1944 to promote good sanitation. Its main goal is to bring together experts in public health, manufacturing, and sanitation. These experts come from government, industry, academia, and public backgrounds to develop and administer performance standards for products that have some impact on sanitation and public health. NSF maintains state-of-the-art laboratories where products can be tested according to the standards they establish. Manufacturers voluntarily submit products for evaluation. If the products pass the tests, then they are *listed* and certain tested claims are *certified*. The certified products are now authorized to display the NSF/ANSI seal on their labels and literature. Although non-governmental, NSF International does have the status as the lead agency for testing and approving the chemicals used in water treatment plants and the materials of construction used in drinking water systems. It earned this status because of its contract with the U.S. Environmental Protection Agency.

The American National Standards Institute (ANSI) and its European equivalent, the Dutch Council for Certification (RVC) recognize NSF International standards. The ANSI is a private, non-profit corporation founded in 1918 for the purpose of enhancing the "global competitiveness of U.S. business and the American quality of life by promoting and facilitating voluntary consensus standards."[1] NSF International's reputation for thoroughness, independence and credibility has made it one of the most trusted public agencies in the world. This well-known corporation has also received the distinction of being appointed a registrar for the International Standards Organization (ISO) and a World Health Organization (WHO) Collaborating Center for Water Safety and Treatment.

There are two NSF International/ANSI Standards for *Drinking Water Treatment Units* (not including others for reverse osmosis, ion exchange, and ultra-violet units): Standard 42 for Aesthetic Effects and Standard 53 for Health Effects. These standards are similar with most of the basic requirements the same for both. A water filter that is "NSF-Listed' or has claims that it is "NSF-Certified" has these qualifications.

---

1. It's been thoughtfully designed and carefully constructed.
   A. It uses established water treatment media and methods.
   B. Its construction materials are tested and documented to be appropriate for potable water use.
   C. The filter is tested and verified to conform to minimum standards of mechanical and hydraulic strength.
   D. It is also tested and verified to conform to minimum standards of hydraulic functioning (minimum flow rate, maximum initial pressure drop, reasonable freedom from channeling and dumping).
2. It has been adequately and truthfully labeled and advertised.
3. It is routinely re-tested. Its manufacturing procedures, documentation and facilities are inspected and audited annually.
4. In addition to the above good manufacturing practices required of all listed products, it's been tested and approved for one or more specific functions that are required to be listed immediately next to the NSF International seal on labels and literature.

Water filters with a Standard 42 (aesthetic effects) certification are designed solely to minimize non-health related contaminants, such as chlorine, taste and odor, and particulates. These filters sorted by classes of performance. For all other claims, there is only a pass or fail.
For taste and odor, each class represents chlorine reduction efficiency.
   Class I, a minimum of 75% chlorine reduction.
   Class II, 50% reduction.
   Class III, 25%.
For mechanical filtration, each class represents particle size ranges that are removed with a minimum 85% efficiency.
   Class I, ½ -1 micron.
   Class II, 1-5 microns.
   Class III, 5-15 microns.
   Class IV, 15-30 microns.

Class V, 30-50 microns.

Class VI, 50+ microns.

Class I or Class II rating does not imply cyst reduction. In order for a water filter to qualify for cyst (parasite) reduction, it must have a 99.95 % minimum filtration efficiency for 3-4-micron test dust particles, 3.000 micron micro-spheres, or live cryptosporidium oocysts.

Water filters with a Standard 53 (health effects) certification are meant to reduce health-related contaminants that may be present in public or private drinking water. Filters that meet the Standard 53 requirements are able to minimize exposure to microbiological, chemical, or particulate contaminants that might be hazardous to your health. These types of filters are typically best suited for individuals who have well water. Some filters fall under the scope of both abovementioned standards since they meet aesthetic and health related claims.

Multipure™ Drinking Water Systems is the only company that produces filters certified and tested according to NSF/ANSI Standards 42 (aesthetics), 53 (Health Effects) and 401 (Emerging Contaminants) for the reduction of all the following.

- Arsenic
- Asbestos
- Atenolol
- Bisphenol A
- Carbamazephine
- Chloramine
- Chloride
- Cyst (Giardia, Cryptosporidium, Entamoeba, Toxoplasma)
- DEET
- Estrone
- Ibuprophen
- Lead
- Linuron
- Meprobamate
- Mercury
- Metolachlor
- MTBE
- Naproxen

- Nonyl phenol
- Particulate matter, Class I (0.5 micron)
- PCB
- Phenytoin
- Radon
- TCEP
- TCPP
- Toxaphene
- Trimethoprim
- Turbidity
- Volatile Organic Chemicals

Multipure™ is the only company in the world certified by NSF that produces 12 different filters that take out arsenic, pharmaceutical drugs, and other emerging contaminants such as pesticides from the water. Because Multipure™ produces the highest rated filters in the world, this is what I use and recommend for family, friends, and patients.

Reference List

1. American National Standards Institute. *ANSI Standards Activities.* https://www.ansi.org/standards_activities/overview/overview. 2018. Accessed Feb 16, 2018.

Chapter 15: Water Pollution Solutions

My first memory of being aware that the quality of drinking water could impact an individual's health was in my first year of chiropractic school at Logan University Health Sciences in Chesterfield, Missouri in 1977. Someone in my class was talking about fasting and recommended reading the book, *The Miracle of Fasting,* by Paul Bragg. Later that same year I went to a Bio-Energetic Synchronization Technique (B.E.S.T) seminar by a Dr. M. T. Morter, DC, MS, who was a developer of this technique and later became President of both Logan University of Health Sciences and Parker University in Dallas, Texas, two of the top chiropractic colleges in the United States. Dr. Morter was a proponent of drinking distilled water and intermittent fasting as well as alkalizing the body with organic minerals. It was at this time that I began periodic water fasting under his direction.

Early in my career, I often routinely recommended patients drink a gallon per day of distilled water for three days to help relieve all kinds of inflammatory processes—disc problems, tendinitis, gastritis, and the like. Invariably, this recommendation helped in varying degrees in reducing inflammation in most individuals. I can recall reading another book early in my professional career called *Fluoride the Aging Factor: How to Recognize and Avoid the Devastating Effects of Fluoride* by Dr. John Yiamouyiannis. After reading the overwhelming evidence presented in this book, I wondered how any municipality could allow fluoride to be put into the water supply. Since the early 1980s when I first read this book, there has been an irrefutable amount of scientific evidence demonstrating the multiple dangers of fluoride toxicity, yet ignorance and denial still abound on this subject. I also became aware of how political certain health issues are when a colleague of mine, who had a long-standing radio show on nutrition, had his show cancelled after having a guest who spoke out against the fluoridation of water in the community.

Reverse Osmosis

In 1983, I purchased a small tabletop reverse osmosis unit that connected directly to the kitchen sink and held one gallon of water. The reverse osmosis unit was less expensive and less cumbersome than a personal distiller. I soon began retailing these to my patients for $199. Pure water has always been part of a foundational program for improving the health of my patients. The only negative aspect of distilled and reverse osmosis water is that both methods remove good minerals along with the toxins like chlorine and fluoride in the water. Therefore, mineral supplementation is necessary. Mineral supplementation is necessary for everyone even without drinking distilled or reverse osmosis water because of the decreased mineral content of food sources. Farming depletes soils of many minerals unless replenished with organic matter. Basically, the longer soil has been farmed the more depleted of minerals it is likely to be. It can take up to 100 years to rebuild the soil after agriculture has been abandoned in a region.[1]

The recommendations of using reverse osmosis drinking water and mineral supplementation have been routine in my practice for 35+ years. In the eighties, I also recommended a green powder product called Green Magma® to my patients to increase their organic mineral intake. Green Magma® is dehydrated organic barley sprouts developed by a Japanese researcher, Dr. Yoshida Hagiwara. Today, there are tens of these organic green powder drinks in the marketplace.

ERW (electrolyzed reduced water)

In 2010, I became aware of a new process that uses electrolysis to release hydrogen ions in the water to varying degrees to make water more bio-available. The process mimics nature and causes the water to be negatively charged, which allows for better hydration. The Japanese conducted extensive research on this technology.[3] The Kangen water system came out of this research. In 2003, Dr. Peter Agre was awarded the Nobel Prize for discovering the positively charged water channels in the cells. He called these water channels the *aquaporin*.[3]

Because the water is negatively charged, cells absorb it more readily because of the opposite positively ion charged water channels. It is my assumption that clean naturally occurring water should and would be negatively charged by divine design. Negatively charged water is what is found in deep well water and other natural healing waters on the planet. I used to supply my patients with non-BPA plastic containers so they could drink the water during initial treatment to help reduce inflammation and pain. The patients drank a gallon per day for three days. The vast majority of patients experienced a reduction of pain during this initial 72-hour period, and I observed the same.

Alkaline water is one of the latest trends. Making any water more alkaline in pH has little health benefits in and of itself. I can give you an example of why that is true. I owned a home with a swimming pool for several years. I could add an assortment of different chemicals to it to make it more alkaline, but that didn't mean the water was healthier to drink. The water still contained chlorine and other toxins that were present in the municipality water supply.

Let me explain further. The secret to ERW (electrolyzed reduced water) being a healthier water is not because of the increased alkalinity per se, but in its availability to give up an electron from the hydrogen to help mitigate ROS (reactive oxygen species), aka free radicals. The electrolysis process creates free hydrogen ions temporarily in the water. You may remember that water is H_2O—two hydrogen ions with a valence of +1 each and a single oxygen ion with a valence of -2. Increasing the amount of electrolysis increases the splitting of hydrogen ions and increases the relative alkalinity in the water. ROS are free radicals needing an electron to neutralize them. The H^+ ion binds with the ROS and negates it. Therefore, this type of water is antioxidant water, which means it is anti-inflammatory and anti-aging water.[2]

The ERW (electrolyzed reduced water) mimics NRW (naturally reduced water) found in water sources that come from deep underground through layers of rock. It is thought that the earth's magnetic field causes an electrolysis-like effect, making hydrogen ions available in the form of hydrogen gas in the water. This natural electrolysis process produces a negative charge in the water as demonstrated by an ORP (oxidation reduction potential) meter. This instrument measures the ability of the water to donate an electron of H^+ to reduce oxidation, the ROS (reactive oxygen species) aka free radicals that are thought to cause degenerative aging.

There are at least seven known locations on the planet that have been documented to have water with unusual healing properties. All are naturally reduced waters. Tens of thousands of people make pilgrimages to these locations every year to gain the reputed healing benefits: These locations include Nordenau, Germany; Lourdes, France; Tiacote, Mexico; Nadama, India; Pamukale, Turkey; Liaoning, China; and Kusatsu Onsen, Japan. The Japanese discovered that the secret of the healing water was not alkalinity, but the availability of free hydrogen ions in the water. The electromagnetic field of the earth is the most likely source of the electrolysis-like process. I want to state this again. It is the water's ability to give up a hydrogen ion to an individual that benefits his/her health, not the alkalinity. This ability to give up hydrogen ions is short lived. If this water is bottled and drunk 24 hours later, it loses the free hydrogen gas ions while remaining alkaline. The free hydrogen ions will have diffused back into the water by this time. Therefore, the same healing water located at these seven locations only works for a few hours. This availability of the hydrogen ions is short lived by hours. It should also be borne in mind that those people who were healed bathed in the water and drank about three liters of this water for a period of two to three weeks to get the beneficial effect. It was not instantaneous.

Hydration

Before Dr. Agre discovered the presence of aquaporins, it was thought that all water was absorbed into the cells by osmosis. Cell membranes control the influx of all nutrients into the cells. The cell membrane contains many different receptor sites that work like a lock-key manner to control the influx of nutrients, hormones, and water. This influx or efflux through the cell membrane is associated with an exchange or attraction of opposite polarities. In the case of the aquaporin, the water channel is positively charged. Therefore, negatively charged water, either NRW or ERW is attracted into the positively charged channel. Conversely, positively charged water like tap water, distilled water, reverse osmosis water, and bottled water that is not negatively charged cannot readily enter the cell for proper hydration.

Most of the water we drink is proton rich, oxidizing, and not absorbed into the cell: When Cornell Medical Center conducted a survey of their patients, 3003 were found to be dehydrated.[4] If a cell cannot absorb sufficient water, it cannot function properly or rid itself of the toxic wastes of cellular metabolism. Just consider how much money is spent on sports drinks in an attempt to hydrate properly. In 2013, sports drinks were a $6.9 billion business in the U.S.[5] All sports drinks I have tested with the ORP meter were proton-rich and positively charged. Clean, negatively charged water will out-perform any sports drink for hydration because it is innately designed to work that way. There are at least 12 major league baseball teams that use this electrolyzed reduced water system.[6]

In addition to the previously mentioned locations, negatively charged water can be found in deep well water. However, one problem with well water, and in fact, all water is the potential infiltration of arsenic, pesticides, herbicides, petroleum by-products, and other environmental toxins. As mentioned in Chapter 9: Glyphosates, many patients in my Florida practice have large amounts of this toxic herbicide in their bodies. Glyphosate is especially harmful to young children, causing learning and behavior dysfunctions. Breakfast cereals made from GMO grains have large amounts of glyphosate.

Water Quality

Another factor to consider with water is the quality of the water to be electrically reduced. Recently Mosaic, the manufacturer of phosphorus-based fertilizer headquartered in Florida accidentally introduced hundreds of millions of gallons of radioactive water into the underground aquifer.[7] After living for 62 years, I feel strongly that each person needs to take her/his own responsibility to learn the facts about water quality. Water pollution is more common in the U.S. than many people know. A three-year EPA study of tap water in 45 states found 316 separate contaminants. This included the 114 contaminants currently regulated and an additional 202 non-regulated ones.[8] Foods, drugs, cosmetics, and pesticides are exempt from the Toxic Substances Control Act. Additionally, cysts (parasites), lead, mercury, asbestos, MTBEs, VOCs, PCBs, chloramine, and arsenic are found in US tap water. Fortunately, the (2015) NSF/ANSI Standard '401' Water Filter Certification guarantees the removal of prescription and OTC medications, herbicides, pesticides, and other emerging chemicals that are not removed in municipal water treatment.

Many people use a single-granulated carbon filter, which is inadequate to reduce significantly or eliminate the many environmental toxins in water. As an alternative, many people drink bottled water with questionable quality. Although reverse osmosis water is available in plastic bottles, I have concerns regarding the plastic bottles themselves. My best recommendation is to buy a carbon block technology with the formal 2015 NSF/ANSI Standard '401' Water Filter Certification, which is the highest rating a water filter can receive. A filter with this rating eliminates arsenic and pharmaceutical drugs. There are currently only three states in the U.S.—California, Wisconsin, and Idaho—that mandate water filtration manufacturers use NSF to market and sell their products. Not understanding this rating makes it difficult for consumers to understand the true capabilities of any particular water filtration system.

I was not aware of NSF until recently but now that I know that this rating exists it is my new "gold standard" for determining what system I use at home and the office and for my patients. The system that I use and recommend is the *aquaperform* made by Multipure[TM]. It is the only manufacturer that has been tested and approved at the highest level of removing arsenic and pharmaceuticals. It comes on the counter top or under the counter top versions. Unfortunately, if you live in or near a larger municipality, you could be consuming pharmaceuticals in your drinking water. An Associated Press investigation found a wide array of prescribed substances in municipal drinking water of 50 cities and in watersheds. The article notes that reverse osmosis will eliminate these toxins.[9] There are currently no national standards regarding safe levels of pharmaceuticals in drinking water.

As discussed earlier in the book, drugs are active at just a few ppb and can produce dangerous side effects at these levels. At the very least, their presence places an ever-increasing body burden of toxicity on the liver. For these reasons, I recommend the Multipure[TM] water filtration systems.

For electrically reduced water systems, I have found the Living Water system produced by Vollara[TM] to be the most trouble-free, well-engineered, aesthetically pleasing, and affordable. They have a patented electrolysis plate that self-cleans. In addition, it contains a regulator to assure the same volume of water comes in contact with the electrolysis plate. The regulator adjusts for varying mineral content of the water so that the amount of electrical charge is consistent to assure the same hydrogen ion and pH production despite varying water sources in different geographic locations. At my clinic, I recommend all patients clean the water first with the Multipure™ and then use the Living Water system to assure the most pristine, anti-oxidant drinking water possible.

Vollara™ also manufactures LaundryPure, a device that acidifies the water and makes hydrogen peroxide, allowing dirty clothes to be cleaned in cold water without laundry detergent and fabric softener. Not only are the clothes and linens clean, but they also contain no residual petroleum by-products to be absorbed transdermally. This process further reduces more environmental toxins and reduces the likelihood of skin contact dermatitis and rashes. Ultimately, it reduces the cost of doing laundry and is a green technology.

Reference List

1. Foster D, Swanson F, Aber J et.al. The importance of land-use legacies to ecology and conservation. *BioScience* 2003 Jan; 53(1): 77-88. doi: 10.1641/0006-3568(2003)053[0077:TIOLUL]2.0.CO;2.
2. Shirahata S, Hamasaki T, Teruya K. Advance research on the health benefit of reduced water. *Trends in Food Science & Technology* 2012 Feb; 23(2): 124-131. doi: 10.1016/j.tifs.2011.10.009.
3. Knepper MA, Nielsen S. Peter Agre, 2003 Nobel Prize winner in chemistry. *J Am Soc Nephrol* 2004 Apr; 15(4): 1093-1095. https://www.ncbi.nlm.nih.gov/pubmed/15034115. Accessed Feb 21, 2018.
4. Meyerowitz S. *Water-the ultimate cure: discover why water is the most important ingredient in your diet and find out which water is right for you.* Summerton, TN: Book Pub Co. 2001.
5. Warmoth B. Sports drinks: a $6.9 B market—and it's only getting bigger. *Food Dive* 2013 Oct 10. https://www.fooddive.com/news/sports-drinks-a-69b-

marketand-its-only-getting-bigger/180655/. Accessed Feb 21, 2018.
6. Vollara. *Proof Book: essential support and validation for Vollara's science and technology, 2nd edition.* https://www.leiaryan.net/uploads/8/1/9/9/8199819/vpb_volla ra_proof_book.pdf. Accessed Apr 16, 2018.
7. CBS/AP. *Fertilizer plant leak leads to massive sinkhole in Florida.* Sept 16, 2016. https://www.cbsnews.com/news/fertilizer-plant-leak-leads-to-massive-sinkhole-in-florida/. Accessed Feb 21, 2018.
8. Luntz T. US drinking water highly contaminated: EPA finds 202 unregulated chemicals in 45 states. *Scientific American* 2009 Dec 14. https://www.scientificamerican.com/article/tap-drinking-water-contaminants-pollutants/. Accessed Feb 17, 2018.
9. Donn J, Mendoza M, Pritchard J. *Pharmawater I: pharmaceuticals found in drinking water, affecting wildlife and maybe humans.* http://hosted.ap.org/specials/interactives/pharmawater_site/da y1_01.html. Accessed Feb 22, 2018.

Since World War II, over 80,000 chemicals, many of which are known carcinogens and endocrine disruptors that cause learning and behavioral problems, have been synthesized. More than four billion pounds of these chemicals are released into the environment through the air, water, food, and household and personal products. The EPA or any governmental agency has not adequately tested the vast majority to evaluate the safety or effects on humans.[1]

There are three primary ways in which air pollutants have a negative impact on bodies. First, air pollution in the form of fine particulates causes an imbalance in the autonomic nervous system imbalance with sympathetic dominance (fight/flight response).[2] The autonomic nervous system regulates cardiac functions,[3-4] digestion, and healing. Autonomic dysfunction of sympathetic dominance leads to a decreased heart rate variability or less variation in the time intervals between heart beats, a condition that is associated with increased cardiac mortality. Many people think that heart rates should be steady. The truth is the greater the amount of heart variability the better.

Second, environmental pollutants harm bodies by causing an overproduction of reactive oxygen and nitrogen species, aka free radicals.[5-6] Inhaling these tiny particles induces tremendous antioxidant stress on the body, exhausting glutathione and super oxide dismutase reserves. Without these protective substances, the liver cannot keep up with detoxification and prevent injury to mitochondria, this condition contributing to a range of chronic diseases from cancer to premature aging.

Third, air pollution increases body-wide inflammation.[7-8] Increased air pollution correlates to increased blood levels of inflammatory chemical messengers called cytokines.[9]

Autonomic Nervous System Problems

There are a number of studies chronicling the effects of air pollution on the autonomic nervous system, particularly in terms of cardiovascular episodes. Those mentioned here are just a sampling. During winter of 1984/1985, 2681 people ages 25 to 64 years old participated in the MONICA Augsburg survey. When these same people were surveyed two years later, there had been an increased acceleration of heartbeats by 1.8 beats per minute during air pollution episodes.[10] A clinical study in 2010 confirmed the correlation between air pollution and heart dysfunction with increased cardiac deaths when atmospheric pollution increased.[11] Similar results are repeated in other studies.[2]

Overproduction of Free Radicals and Resulting Inflammation

As with air pollution and autonomic nervous system problems, there is a plethora of studies regarding air pollution creating oxidative stress that results in inflammation. Consequences of this include lung inflammation,[12] lung cancer, acute respiratory infections,[14] and asthmatic attacks.[13] Additional conditions related to free radical damage caused by air pollution include emphysema, cardiovascular and inflammatory diseases, and cataracts.[15]

Chronic exposure to air pollution takes a cumulative toll on the body's defenses and is linked to the increasing incidence of many insidious diseases of recent history: cardiovascular and chronic respiratory disease,[3,4,7] glucose intolerance,[5] premature births among asthmatic mother,[6] ulcerative colitis[16], kidney disease[17], thyroid disease[18], decreased heart rate variability[20], impaired lung function[22,23], lung and other cancers[19,23,24], impaired cognitive function[25], asthma exacerbation[22], increase mortality[26], and reduced life expectancy.[27-32] Air pollution is also responsible for loss of quality of life and longevity. Exposure to toxic particles is associated with increased rates of cardiovascular and respiratory illness and death.[3,4] New studies have demonstrated damage occurring to blood vessels of individuals as young as age 23.[7] According to researchers from MIT (Massachusetts Institute of Technology) air pollution is responsible for his many as 200,000 premature deaths each year in this United States.[1]

Sources of Exposure

Air pollutants are divided into two classes denoted by size. Fine particulates are high risk particles denoted by the sign $PM_{2.5}$ and are less than 2.5 microns in diameter. PM_{10}, the larger particles, can travel through the bronchioles of the lung to the alveoli and enter the bloodstream, causing damage to the endothelium of the blood vessels and many other critical body functions.[20-22] To put the size of these particles into a better perspective, a human hair is about 70 microns in diameter.[20] Air pollution has become a serious global health epidemic. Approximately 80% of the people on the planet live in areas where the air pollution exceeds World Health Organization air quality guidelines.[33]

In 2009, the CDC investigated the level of the accumulation of toxins (body burden) in the U.S. population for some 212 industrial chemicals and found high levels of many of the more common chemicals, including PBDE (polybrominated diphenyl ethers) and BPA (Bisphenol A), which are endocrine disruptors, adversely affecting reproduction.[14] Perfluoroalkyl 15, a member of the PFOAO (perfluro-octanoic acid) chemical family, that has been linked to diseases ranging from kidney disease to cancer,[16-19] was found in 98% of those tested. The overheating of Teflon[TM] coated pans can release these fumes.

Another source of ongoing and cumulative body burden of environmental toxins is the air we breathe on a daily basis at home or work. Indoor pollution in the 200-500% more polluted than outdoor. People spend 90% of their time indoors. Energy efficient homes and buildings trap pollutants.[34] Allergic reactions, asthma triggers, headaches, eye irritation, coughing, dizziness, sore throat, nasal discharge, airway constriction, shortness of breath and wheezing are some of the common symptoms caused by indoor air pollution. At least 1 in 3 families suffer from multiple signs and symptoms of indoor pollution. Pharmaceutical companies net $10 billion each year providing solutions in this country that only mask the symptoms. When was the last time your doctor or physician asked you to test the quality of the air you were breathing?

Sources of indoor air pollution are mold and mildew, ragweed and pollen, tobacco smoke, pets and dander, dust, outside air, and chemicals in household products. The chemical scents and fragrances can contain between 100 and 350 different chemicals. Breathing these chemicals adversely affects asthma sufferers and causes others to display many of the above-mentioned symptoms.[35.]

What You Can Do

Although you cannot avoid air pollution, you can greatly reduce the amount in your home and office by using NASA approved technologies like Active Pure. I use the Active Pure air scrubbing systems in my home and office and take a mobile unit with me when I travel to place in the hotel room. This greatly improves the quality of the air by removing or reducing the many contaminants negatively impacting health.

The air scrubber produces antioxidant air. One of the most damaging effects of air pollution is the increase of oxidative stress on the body. [26-32,36] When I place the ORP meter up to the air scrubber and surrounding air space, a negative reading appears on the meter indicating that the air is donating electrons that can bind to ROS (reactive oxygen species) aka free radicals.

Specific nutrients aid in inhibiting the adverse effects of the air pollutants and facilitate the removal of them from the body. Omega-3 fatty acids have demonstrated the ability to increase the body's natural defenses and combat oxidative stress.[31-32,36] One group of older people received 2 grams of Omega 3 PUFA (polyunsaturated fatty acid from fish oil) to evaluate its potential impact on the oxidative stress response to $PM_{2.5}$ particles over a period of 4 months. This high dose created a 49% increase in super oxide dismutase activity, which equates to increased protection of cell and mitochondria membranes.[37] There was an additional 62% increase in glutathione (GSH) that equated to an increase ability of the liver to detoxify[4] and a 72% decrease in lipid peroxidation that equated to increased protection of vascular endothelial and cell membrane. All these markers indicate a high activity of endogenous antioxidants.[37] In another study, non-symptomatic middle-aged individuals received 3 grams of omega-3 fish oil daily for a three-week period. They were exposed to concentrated ambient fine and ultrafine particles. The researchers found that the omega-3s effectively blocked negative cardio-lipid effects caused by the particulate pollutants.[38]

The EPA compared the consumption of 3 grams of omega 3s or olive oil versa a control group that did not receive these supplements. Forty-two subjects received either 3 grams of omega-3s or 3 grams of olive oil every day for a month. A third group served as a control and received neither. A baseline was established by having the participants exposed to 2 hours of filtered air. On the second day, they were exposed to 2 hours of fine and ultrafine concentrated ambient particulate matter, a dangerous component of air pollution. To measure the difference, the endothelial function of each individual was tested by measuring the flow-mediated dilation of the brachial artery. I also do this evaluation.

Additional testing was done by measuring each subject's fibrinolysis, the body's natural anti-clotting activity. If you are on Coumadin, this test is done routinely to evaluate the prothrombin time in your blood work.

Of the two supplements, it was found the olive oil seemed to have given better protection than the omega-3s in preserving the ability of the blood vessels to dilate. As to be expected the control group experienced a significantly reduced flow-mediated dilation.[39] In addition, the olive oil group maintained elevated levels of plasminogen actides, a protein that breaks down blood clots for twenty hours after exposure to the polluted air. [39] Both the omega-3s and olive oil helped maintain the blood vessels ability to dilate. However, the olive oil had better performance in reducing blood clots. Recalling the seven sequela of stress in the first chapter, the olive oil seemed to better inhibit the sympathetic (fight/flight) response by flight spots that causes constriction of the blood vessels and provide better protection of the endothelium and better reduction of the stickiness of the red blood cells and platelets.

Compounds in cruciferous vegetables, such as broccoli, cauliflower, Brussel sprouts, kale, and water cress, also protect against the harmful effects of air pollution. Unpregulated sulfurphane (enhanced so that more will be absorbed), a compound found in broccoli, contain enzymes that help to combat oxidative stress in the upper respiratory tract. Broccoli brown extract containing a sulfuphane precursor has been found to reduce nasal allergic responses to diesal exhaust particulates.[40] Cruciferous vegetables facilitate the detoxification of airborne pollutants, including benzene which is extremely carcinogenic41, and assist both phase I and phase II liver detoxification pathways.

Glucosinolate in Brussels sprouts can reduce the oxidative DNA damage caused by toxins by up to 28%. This component reduces the carcinogenic potential of environmental toxins by increasing the genetic expression of critical detoxifying enzymes.[42,43] Water cress also contains a derivative of glucosinolate that protects against DNA damage.[44,45] The water cress extract protects against high risk carcinogens found in tobacco smoke.[44-46]

121

Individuals with a lower intake of folate, B6, and B12 show significantly reduced heart rate variability 48 hours after being exposed to increased $PM_{2.5}$ levels.[47] However, in those individuals with high daily dietary intake of these protective nutrients, the negative effects of a small particulate pollution on heart rate variability was prevented. A decreased heart rate variability indicates a dominant sympathetic nervous system and is indicative of reduced longevity. It is important to remember that these three B vitamin and riboflavin are interdependent upon each other for absorption and are used in thousands of enzyme processes in the body. This is just one of many reasons B vitamin supplementation is a must for optimal health in today's world.

The old standby antioxidants Vitamin C and Vitamin E have been found effective and work synergistically to protect the body from oxidative stress caused by air pollution. A study in Brazil measured oxidative stress bio-markers before and after supplementation. One group was exposed to coal-burning emissions from a power plant before and after supplementation of 500 mg of Vitamin C and 800 IU of Vitamin E. Those receiving supplements were then compared to a control group of non-exposed individuals. After 6 months, the bio-markers were re-measured. Individuals who were exposed to the air pollution before supplementation demonstrated significant decreased levels of key protective substances such as glutathione and Vitamin E and demonstrated impairment of antioxidant enzymes including catalase, glutathione peroxidase, glutathione reductase, and glutathione-S-transferase. Additionally, the markers for lipid and protein damage increased.[48]

After the exposed group was supplemented with Vitamin C and Vitamin E for 6 months, they were retested. The markers for lipid and protein damage decreased and antioxidant defenses were comparable to the levels of the group that was not exposed.[48]

Other studies have shown benefits from supplementing a combination of Vitamin C and Vitamin E on asthma patients.[48,50] They have been shown to reduce ozone associated lung function decline[49] and ozone induced bronchial hyperresponsiveness.[50] Air pollution has a direct negative impact on the ability of the individual to produce Vitamin D from sun exposure. Air pollution reduces the amount of ultraviolet-B (UVB) radiation that reaches the ground level and subsequently your skin.

In one study, Vitamin D levels of residents of rural areas were compared to residents of a polluted urban area. The serum levels of 25-hydroxyvitamin D (25 (OH)D) were compared in two groups. It was found that the residents living in the polluted urbans areas needed two to three times the *sun exposure index* to obtain comparable levels of those living in the rural area.

Children living in the more polluted part of Deli, India, had mean serum 25(OH)D levels 54% lower than the children living in areas of the city less polluted.[51] In Iran, women living in the polluted city of Tehran were compared to those living in less polluted Ghazvim. The women in Tehran exhibited significantly lower Vitamin D levels. This is an interesting study because it encompasses a study of largely Muslim women who get no sun exposure due to customary dress.[52]

Because the vast majority of people in the U.S. spend 90% of their time indoors, everyone needs to supplement with vitamin D3. I recommend a combination of the D3/K2 for best results. Vitamin D acts as a hormone and is critical in all cellular functions. Every cell in the body has a Vitamin D receptor. Individuals below 19 have an increased risk for all morbidity from cancer, heart disease, diabetes, kidney disease, and the like, related to obesity.[53] Obesity rates for 12 to 19 years of age have increased from 5% to 18%.[54] Decreased Vitamin D levels are associated with obesity.

My Program

In my office, I provide patients with petri dishes they can take home to test for bacteria or mold overgrowth. In Florida, the majority of the people I test have mold problems in their homes. I also test for body burden of mold in the body through Great Plains Labs. As a solution, I recommend ActivePure™ Technology to my patients. It is a NASA approved technology used in the space station. It converts oxygen and humidity into powerful oxidizers called hydroxyls, destroying microorganisms in the air and surfaces, killing most pathogens on contact. If it is safe for the astronauts in the space station, it is safe for you.

The following are a few studies demonstrating the efficacy of this technology. I have reviewed twenty plus studies on this technology and the results are impressive. The following graphs have been supplied by Vollara™, an offspring of Electrolux.

The Kansas State test results graph shown below demonstrates an average reduction of multiple microbes—bacteria, virus, and mold—in the air and surface by 80% within 2 hours, 95% within 6 hours, and 99% within 24 hours with the ActivePure™ technology.

Vollara™ Graph 1

Testing by Kansas State University

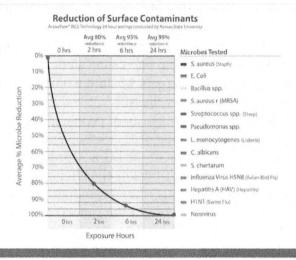

The graph below shows the reduction of particles in a residential setting.

Vollara™ Graph 2

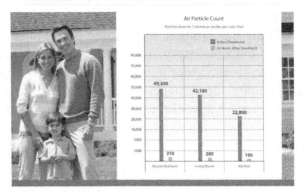

Vollara^{TM} graph 3 below shows a major operating room study. It demonstrates a 90.1 % reduction in air particulates under .1 micron in one day, 83.4 % reduction in bacteria count, and 95.7 % reduction in MRSA combined in day 1 and 2 of testing.

Vollara^{TM} Graph 3

Major Hospital Operating Room Results – **Elimination!**

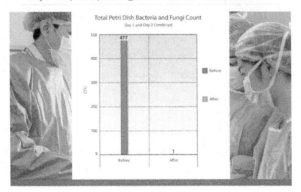

The Vollara^{TM} Graph 4 shows the results of a study conducted at an Indiana education facility. The two bars on the left represent the number of flu related dismissals from school. In the first month, there were 40. By the third month, there were 118. During the fourth month, half of the air purification units were installed using the ActivePure^{TM} technology. By month five, flu related dismissals were down to 13, where they remained through month 10 when the other half of the ActivePure™ systems were installed. By month 13, there were only 8 cases.

   To bring this problem into a more personal context I submit the following anecdotal story. We have a younger associate at the clinic who exercises regularly, eats a better than average diet, and takes good quality supplements. However, she suffered a respiratory--type illness every 4-6 weeks, causing her to miss a day of work. Shortly after we began using this air filtration system in the office she took one of the test kits home to test the air quality in her apartment.

Vollara™ Graph 4

Education Facility - Indiana

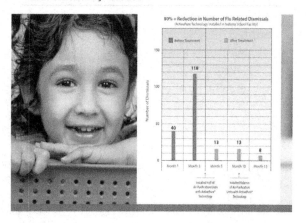

Week 1 Petri Dish Results

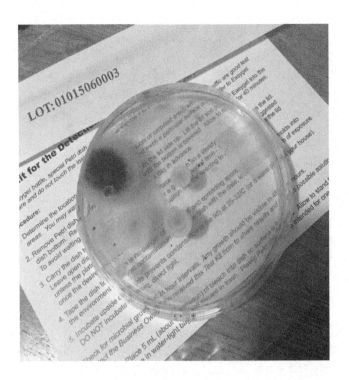

She then used an ozone air cleaner for a week and re-tested.

Week 2 Petri Dish results

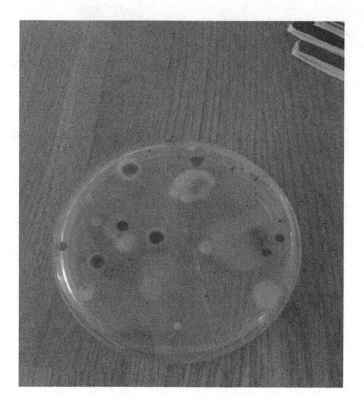

As you can see the ozone did not do much. If anything, it might look a little worse. After this she took home the same air scrubber with the NASA approved technology I use in the office and recommend to patients.

Petri Dish Results after NASA approved technology

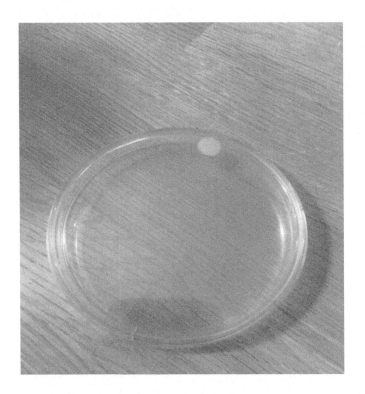

There had been a water leak in the apartment several months earlier causing the mold growth. This apartment needed to have the mold treated but in the meantime the air scrubber was taking the vast majority of the mold out of her breathing space. This was in June 2016, and she hasn't been ill since February, 2017, and she has had no more respiratory illnesses, nausea, or vomiting and has missed no work. How many of you are experiencing similar problems and looking in the wrong direction for solutions? Although medications are absolutely necessary and life-saving in certain emergencies, there are very few that do not cause side effects if taken long enough. More importantly, medications are not treating the cause of this type problem. I had a pharmacist tell me once that there is no prescription medication taken long enough that will not cause its own illness/disease.

In a study conducted by the University of Cincinnati,[55] the ActivePure[TM] Technology reduced 90% of the pathogens in the air in just 30 minutes. This is 50 times more powerful than normal HVAC filtrations. Another great thing I love about the machine is that there are no replacement filters. The air filter is cleaned about once per month by simply removing one screw and panel. The air scrubber even prompts you with a message when it needs to be cleaned. See the University of Cincinnati study below.

Vollara™ Graph 5

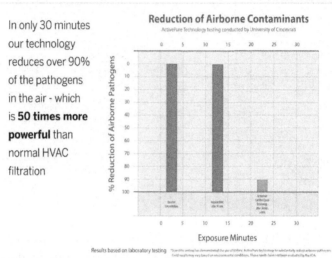

How Powerful is ActivePure Technology?
University of Cincinnati Reduction of Airborne Pathogens

In only 30 minutes our technology reduces over 90% of the pathogens in the air - which is **50 times more powerful** than normal HVAC filtration

Reduction of Airborne Contaminants
ActivePure Technology testing conducted by University of Cincinnati

Results based on laboratory testing

There are multiple benefits of fresher, cleaner air from using the ActivePure™ Technology.
1. Reduction in sick days and the number of common cold and flu outbreaks.
2. Protection from common and reoccurring allergy and asthma triggers.
3. Removes volatile organic compounds.
4. Reduction in respiratory illnesses.
5. Improved productivity from healthier air and surfaces.
6. Protection from illness causing bacteria and viruses such as MRSA and E. Coli.
7. Odor control.
8. Better sleep.

The use of this technology is one of the tools I use in my practice to help my patients to reduce their body burden of airborne contaminants. I have often loaned a unit to a patient over the weekend, and each has experienced so much improvement in breathing, sinus congestion, cough, and sleeping within 48-72 hours that the patient arranges to purchase one.

One of the best ways to improve air quality and greatly reduce the number of negative particles in the air is to use the ActivePure™ System air technology. This is what I use in my home and office, when I am traveling, and what I recommend to all my patients. Information about these systems is available on my website: www.drkellymiller.com. Please call the office at 813-985-1322 if you have any questions about how to obtain such a system.

Reference List

1. Mount Sinai Children's Environmental Health Center. *New York states Children and the Environment.* https://www.mountsinai.org/static_files/MSMC/Files/Patient%20Care/Children/Childrens%20Environmental%20Health%20Center/NYS-Children-Environment.pdf. Dec, 2013. Accessed Feb 23, 2018.
2. Middlekauff HR, Park J, Moheimani RS. Adverse effects of cigarette and noncigarette exposure on the autonomic nervous system: mechanisms and implications for cardiovascular risk. *Jour of the Am Coll of Cardiology* 2014 Oct 21; 64(16): 1740-1750. doi: 10.1016/j.jacc.2014.06.1201.
3. Brook RD. Cardiovascular effects of air pollution. *Clin Sci (Lond).* 2008;115(6):175-87. doi: 10.1042/CS20070444.
4. Peters A. Particulate matter and heart disease: evidence from epidemiological studies. *Toxicol Appl Pharmacol.* 2005;207(2 Suppl):477-82.
5. Al-Gubory KH. Environmental pollutants and lifestyle factors induce oxidative stress and poor prenatal development. *Reprod Biomed Online* 2014 Jul; 29(1): 17-31. doi: 10.1016/j.rbmo.2014.03.002.
6. Migliore L, Coppedé F. Environmental-induced oxidative stress in neurodegenerative disorders and aging. *Mutation Research/Genetic Toxicology and Environmental Mutagenesis*

2009 Mar; 674 (1-3): 73-84. doi: 10.1016/j.mrgentox.2008.09.013.

7. Wolf K, Popp A, Schneider A et al. Association between long-term exposure to air pollution and biomarkers related to insulin resistance, subclinical inflammation, and adipokines. *Diabetes.* 2016;65(11):3314-26. https://www.ncbi.nlm.nih.gov/pubmed/27605624. Accessed Feb 23, 2018.

8. Pope CA, 3rd, Bhatnagar A, McCracken JP et al. Exposure to fine particulate air pollution is associated with endothelial injury and systemic inflammation. *Circ Res.* 2016;119(11):1204-1214. https://www.ncbi.nlm.nih.gov/pubmed/27780829. Accessed Feb 23, 2018.

9. van Eden SF, Tan WC, Suwa T et.al. Cytokines involved in the systematic inflammatory response induced by exposure to particulate matter air pollutants (PM(10)). *Am J Respir Crit Care Med* 2001 Sep 1; 16(5): 826-30. https://www.ncbi.nlm.nih.gov/pubmed/11549540. Accessed Feb 23, 2018.

10. Peters A, Perz S, Doring A, Stieber W, Whichman HE. Activation of the autonomic nervous system and blood coagulation in association with air pollution episode. *Inhalation Technology* 2000 Jan; Sup 2-51-61. doi: 10.1080/08958378.2000.11463199.

11. Barthelemy J. Impact of air pollution on the autonomic nervous system activity and the presence of sleep apnea in older subjects (POLLAIR). ClinicalTrials.gov Identifier: NCT01042834. Jan 13, 2011. https://clinicaltrials.gov/ct2/show/NCT01042834. Accessed Feb 23, 2018.

12. Li XY, Gilmour S, Donaldson K, MacNee W. Free radical activity and pro-inflammatory effects of particulate air pollution (PM 10) in vivo and in vitro. *Thorax* 51(2). doi: 10.1136/thx.51.12.1216.

13. Kampa M, Castanas E. Human health effects of air pollution. *Environmental Pollution* 2008 Jan; 151(2): 362-367. 10.1016/j.envpol.2007.06.012.

14. Kelly FJ. Oxidative stress: its role in air pollution and adverse health effects. *Occup and Environ Med* 2003 Aug; 60(8). doi: 10.1136/oem.60.8.612.

15. Machlin LJ, Bendich A. Free radical tissue damage: protective role of antioxidant nutrients. *FASEB Journal* 1987 Dec 1. doi: 10.1096/fasebj.1.6.3315807.

16. Mendola P, Wallace M, Hwang BS, et al. Pretenn birth and air pollution: Critical windows of exposure for women with asthma. *J Allergy Clin Jrn Imunol.* 2016;138(2):432-435.

17. Lloyd-Smith M, Sheffield-Brotherton B. Children's environmental health: intergenerational equity in action—a civil society perspective. *Ann NY Acad Sci.* 2008; 1140:190-200.

18. Environmental Protection Agency. *EPA orders Oahu sugar to begin clean up investigation at Wiapio Peninsula pesticide mixing site.* Mar 30, 2005. https://archive.epa .gov/epapages/newsroom_archive/ newsreleases/c36c6bee520812d585257af5007b9e98.html. Accessed February 24, 2017.

19. Crews D, Gore AC. Epigenetic synthesis: a need for a new paradigm for evolution in a contaminated world. *FIOOO Biol Rep.* 2012; 4:18. http://www.worldometers.info/view/toxchem/. Accessed February 27, 2017.

20. Miller MR. The role of oxidative stress in the cardiovascular actions of particular te air pollution. *Biochem Soc Trans* 2014;42(4):1006-11. doi: 10.1042/BST20140090.

21. Park SK, O'Neill MS, Wright RO, et al. HFE genotype, particulate air pollution, and heart rate variability: a gene-environment inter- action. *Circulation.* 2006;114(25):2798-805. https://www.ncbi.nlm.nih.gov/pubmed/17145987. Accessed March 14, 2018.

22. Oftedal B, Brunekreef B, Nystad W, et al. Residential outdoor air pollution and lung function in schoolchildren. *Epidemiology.* 2008;19(1):129-37. doi: 10.1097/EDE.0b013e31815c0827.

23. Pope CA, 3rd, Burnett RT, Thun MJ, et al. Lung cancer, cardiopulmonary mortality, and long-term exposure to fine particulate air pollution. *Jama.* 2002;287(9):1132-41.

https://www.ncbi.nlm.nih.gov/pubmed/11879110. Accessed Mar 15, 2018.

24. Raaschou-Nielsen O, Andersen ZJ, Beelen R, et al. Air pollution and lung cancer incidence in 17 European cohorts: prospective analyses from the European Study of Cohorts for Air Pollution Effects (ESCAPE). *Lancet Oncol* 2013;14(9):813- 22. doi: 10.1016/S1470-2045(13)70279-1.

25. Ranft U, Schikowski T, Sugiri D et al. Long-term exposure to traffic-related particulate matter impairs cognitive function in the elderly. *Environ Res.* 2009;109(8):1004-11.

26. Hoek G, Brunekreef B, Goldbohm S et al. Association between mortality and indicators of traffic-related air pollution in the Netherlands: a cohort study. *Lancet* 2002; 360(9341):1203-9.

27. Pope CA, 3rd, Ezzati M, Dockery DW. Fine-particulate air pollution and life expectancy in the United States. *N Engl J Med.* 2009;360(4):376-86.

28. Chen Y, Ebenstein A, Greenstone M et al. Evidence on the impact of sustained exposure to air pollution on life expectancy from China's Huai River policy. *Proc Natl Acad Sci USA.* 2013;110(32):12936-41.

29. Correia AW, Pope CA, 3rd, Dockery DW et al. Effect of air pollution control on life expectancy in the United States: an analysis of 545 U.S. counties for the period from 2000 to 2007. *Epidemiology.* 2013;24(1).23-31.

30. Holguin F, Tellez-Rojo MM, Hernandez M, et al. Air pollution and heart rate variability among the elderly in Mexico City. *Epidemiology.* 2003;14(5):521-7.

31. Poljsak B, Fink R. The protective role of antioxidants in the de- fence against ROS/RNS-mediated environmental pollution. *Oxid Med Cell Longev* 2014; 2014:671539.

32. Nel AE, Diaz-Sanchez D, Li N. The role of particulate pollutants in pulmonary inflammation and asthma: evidence for the involvement of organic chemicals and oxidative stress. *Curr Opin Pulm Med* 2001,7(1) :20-6.

33. Center for Disease Control. *National Report on Human Exposure to Environmental Chemicals.* Jan 2017. https://www.cdc.gov/exposurereport/index.html. Accessed Mar 15, 2018.

---

34. Environmental Protection Agency. *Energy, Weatherization and Indoor Air Quality.* Jan 19, 2018. https://www.epa.gov/indoor-air-quality-iaq/energy-weatherization-and-indoor-air-quality. Accessed Mar 15, 2018.

35. *Breathe.* The Lung Association. Dec 10, 2016. https://www.lung.ca/lung-health/air-quality/indoor-air-quality/scents. Accessed Mar 15, 2018.

36. Fujisawa T. Role of oxygen radicals on bronchial asthma. *Curr Drug Targets Inflamm Allergy* 2005;4(4) :505-9. http://www.ingentaconnect.com/content/ben/cdtia/2005/00000 004/00000004/art00014. Accessed Mar 15, 2018.

37. Romieu I, Garcia-Esteban R, Sunyer J et al. The effect of supplementation with omega-3 polyunsaturated fatty acids on markers of oxidative stress in elderly exposed to PM (2.5). *Environ Health Perspect* 2008;116(9:)1237-42. doi: 10.1289/ehp.10578.

38. Tong H, Rappold AG, Diaz-Sanchez D, et al. Omega-3 fatty acid supplementation appears to attenuate particulate air pollution-induced cardiac effects and lipid changes in healthy middle-aged adults. *Environ Health Perspect* 2012;120(7):952-957.

39. Tong H, Rappold AG, Caughey M, et al. Dietary supplementation with olive oil or fish oil and vascular effects of concentrated ambient particulate matter exposure in human volunteers. *Environ Health Perspect* 2015;123(11):1173-9. doi: 10.1289/ehp.1408988.

40. Riedl MA, Saxon A, Diaz-Sanchez D. Oral sulforaphane increases Phase ll antioxidant enzymes in the human upper airway. *Clin Immunol* 2009;130(3):244-51. doi: 10.1016/j.clim.2008.10.007.

41. Heber D, Li Z, Garcia-Lloret M, et al. Sulforaphane-rich broccoli sprout extract attenuates nasal allergic response to diesel exhaust particles. *Food Funct* 2014;5(1):35-41.

42. Verhagen H, Poulsen HE, Loft S, et al. Reduction of oxidanve DNA-damage in humans by Brussels sprouts. *Carcinogenesis.* 1995;16(4):969-70. https://www.ncbi.nlm.nih.gov/pubmed/7728983. Accessed Mar 16, 2018.

43. Nijhoff WA, Grubben MJ, Nagengast FM, et al. Effects of consumption of Brussels sprouts on intestinal and lymphocytic glutathione S-transferases in humans. *Carcinogenesis.* 1995;16(9):2125-8. https://www.ncbi.nlm.nih.gov/pubmed/7554064. Accessed Mar 16, 2018.

44. Rose P, Faulkner K, Williamson G, et al. 7-Methylsulfinylheptyl and 8-methylsulfinyloctyl isothiocyanates from water- cress are potent inducers of phase II enzymes. *Carcinogenesis.* 2000;21(11):1983-8. https://www.ncbi.nlm.nih.gov/pubmed/11062158. Accessed Mar 16, 2018.

45. Gill CI, Haldar S, Boyd LA, et al. Watercress supplementation in diet reduces lymphocyte DNA damage and alters blood antioxidant status in healthy adults. *AmJ Clin Nutr.* 2007;85(2):504-10.57. https://www.ncbi.nlm.nih.gov/pubmed/17284750. Accessed Mar 16, 2018.

46. Hecht SS, Chung FL, Richie JP, Jr, et al. Effects of watercress consumption on metabolism of a tobacco-specific lung carcinogen in smokers. *Cancer Epidemiol Biomarkers Prev.* 1995;4(8):877-84. https://www.ncbi.nlm.nih.gov/pubmed/8634661. Accessed Mar 16, 2018.

47. Baccarelli A, Cassano PA, Litonjua A, et al. Cardiac autonomic dysfunction: eftects from particulate air pollution and protection by dietary methvl nutrients and metabolic polymorphisms. *Circulation* 2008,117(14):1802-9. doi: 10.1161/CIRCULATIONAHA.107.726067.

48. Possamai FP, Junior SA, Parisotto EB, et al. Antioxidant intervention compensates oxidative stress in blood of subjects exposed to emissions from a coal elcctric-power plant in South Brazil. *Environ Toxicol Pharmacol* 2010;30(2):175-80. doi: 10.1016/j.etap.2010.05.006.

49. Romieu I, Sierra-Monge JJ, Ramirez-Aguilar M, et al. Antioxidant supplementation and lung functions among children with asthma exposed to high levels of air pollutants. *Am J Respir Crit Carn Med.* 2002;166(5):703-9.

50. Trenga CA, Koenig JO, Williams PV. Dietary antioxidants and ozone-induced bronchial hyperresponsiveness in adults with asthma. *Arch Environ Health.* 2001;56(3):242-9. https://www.ncbi.nlm.nih.gov/pubmed/11480500. Accessed Mar 16, 2018.

51. Szabolcs P, Holguin F, Wood LG et.al. Nutritional solutions to reduce risks of negative health impacts of air pollution. *Nutrients* 2015 Dec; 7(12):10398-10416. doi: 10.3390/nu7125539.

52. Hosseinpanah F, Hashemi pour S, Heibatollahi M, Asefzade S, Azizi F. The effects of pollution on vitamin D status in healthy women: a cross sectional study. *BMC Public Health* 2010; 10: 519. doi: 10.1186/1471-2458-10-519.

53. Pi-Sunyer X. The medical risk of obesity. *Postgrad Med* 2009 Nov; 12(16): 21-33. doi:10.3810/pgm.2009.11.2074.

54. *Morbidity and Mortality among Adolescents and Young Adults in the United States.* AstraZeneca Fact Sheet 2011. https://www.jhsph.edu/research/centers-and-institutes/center-for-adolescent-health/_images/_pre-redesign/az/US%20Fact%20Sheet_FINAL.pdf. Accessed Mar 16, 2018.

55. Grinshpun S, Adhikari A, Honda T, et. al. Control of aerosol contaminants in indoor air: combining the particle concentration reduction with microbial inactivation. *Environ Sci Technol* 2007; 41:6-6-612.

Chapter 17: Electromagnetic Frequencies (EMFs)

In the U.S. today, there is a probable avalanche of brain-related problems on both ends of the spectrum. As discussed in previous chapters, an increasing number of children are being diagnosed with ADHD and autism spectrum disorders while Alzheimer's disease is the fastest growing cause of death among the aging. All of these problems can be traced to the some 80,000 plus chemicals that permeate the air, food, and water sources. Equally frightening is the research on EMFs in relationship to ADHD, autism spectrum, and Alzheimer's disease. The increased use of cell phones and WI-FI in homes, schools, and work places is taking a toll on brain health. EMFs (Electromagnetic Frequencies) are one of the most detrimental environmental stressors.

While this book was in press, I was busy finishing the manuscript for the fourth book in the series, *Saving Your Brain: Causes, Prevention, and Reversal of Dementia/Alzheimer's*. As this book you are now reading had not yet gone to press, I decided to add a chapter from the brain book to *Is Your Environment Stressing You Out?*. It is my hope that adding this chapter will serve as a transition from this book to the next.

As of January, 2018, The California Department of Public Health just issued a warning about cell phone overuse. In fact, they recommended minimizing the use of cell phones as much as possible and to keep them away from your body as much as possible. The report, titled, *How to Reduce Exposure of Radiofrequency Energy from Cell Phones*[1], provides this information. "Although the science is still evolving, some laboratory experiments and human health studies have suggested the possibility that long-term, high use of cell phones, may be linked to certain types of cancers and other health effects, including:

- Brain cancer and tumors of the acoustic nerve (needed for hearing and maintaining balance) and salivary glands.
- Lower sperm counts and inactive and less mobile sperm.
- Headaches and effects on learning and memory, hearing, behavior, and sleep."

While the research is in its infancy, I believe these results may be only the tip of the iceberg on the potential negative effects of electrical and magnetic fields on the body and brain. As I discussed in my first book, *13 Secrets to Optimal Aging*, in the chapter on melatonin, electrical fields found in an electrical blanket dramatically reduce melatonin levels. This becomes significant in light of the role that melatonin play in preventing and reversing amyloid beta fibrils. Melatonin is the most powerful anti-oxidant the body produces. The benefits of melatonin as it relates to Alzheimer's disease are contained in the chapter on hormones in this book. The fact that EMFs disrupt sleep is significant in that a lack of sleep increases the risk of Alzheimer's disease.

In addition to disrupting sleep, EMFs may also be endocrine disruptors. The theory that EMFs could cause endocrine disruption is substantiated by a reduction in hormones levels in cows exposed to EMFs.[2, 3] A reduction in sperm count demonstrates EMFs ability to disrupt mitochondrial energy production.[4] Additional research suggests that EMFs may also disrupt hypothalamus-pituitary-gonad axis, hypothalamus-pituitary-thyroid axis, and hypothalamus-pituitary-adrenal axis functions as well. The first book provides good explanations of the functions of these axes. Decreased levels of multiple hormones are noted in Alzheimer's patients.

Although EMFs are not in all likelihood the primary cause of Alzheimer's, there is evidence that they act as a cumulative stressor increasing the risk for occurrence. In fact, it is my position that Alzheimer's is the result of a multitude of factors, most of which are under our individual control and are covered in this book. There are numerous studies linking an increased risk of Alzheimer's to exposure to EMF.[5-15] Many of these studies are older and before the almost ubiquitous use of computers, laptops, tablets, and smart phones and the vast expansion of cell towers and WI-FI. Most of the studies are related to the risks of certain occupations exposed to EMFs.[5-6]

However, there is considerable evidence to support the position that the EMFs from cell phones and Wi-Fi are an even greater threat to brains.[7] Physical bodies, including human bodies, are electrical and electromagnetic. Documentation indicates that multiple different type of electrical frequencies and magnetic fields can either have a positive or negative impact on homeostasis.[8] Specifically, EMFs have been shown to cause suppression of melatonin and increased permeability of the blood-brain barrier and alter the effect of Ca++ binding in neurons.[8] Unfortunately, most of the types of electrical frequencies and magnetic fields we encounter have a negative impact on brain health. As I have stated before, what is bad for the body is bad for the brain and what is bad for the brain is bad for the body. As more research comes forth, the cumulative negative effect on the brain from multiple sources of EMFs are likely to be further confirmed. Here is what we know now.

Overall, the incidence (percentage of occurrence) for Alzheimer's is the same for men and women. However, the prevalence (the actual number of cases) is greater in women simply because women live longer than men. In a Swedish study, 931 dementia-free individuals over the age of 75 were monitored for approximately 7 years. Dementia was diagnosed in 265 subjects, including 202 with Alzheimer's by the end of the time frame. Among men, ELF-MF exposure > 0.2 uT over a lifetime job increased the relative risk by 2.3 for Alzheimer's.[5]

In another study done from 1985 to 1996, 537,692 men and 180,529 women in Sweden were evaluated for Alzheimer's as a primary or contributory cause of death. Four different levels of exposure were used for quantification purposes in the group tested. The risk increased in both men and women with increasing EMF exposure, with a relative risk of 4.0 in the highest exposure group.[6] In the two different studies, the increased risk was 2.3 to 4x as great for developing Alzheimer's if exposed to an occupation that was in the immediate proximity of EMF exposure. These relative risk factors are significant and cumulative. It is a question of which straw (stressor) broke the camel's back.

Here are summaries of three of the top researchers in the area of EMF and Alzheimer's disease (AD).

- In the late 1990s, epidemiological studies in the US and in Sweden were conducted by Dr. Eugene Sobel and colleagues of the USC School of Medicine. They reported a four-fold increase in the risk of AD for people who had worked in occupations with medium to high exposure to EMFs.[10-11]
- Also, in the 1990s, Dr. Maria Feychting of Stockholm Sweden reported the results of her study at the Department of Energy's annual research review in San Antonio, TX. Studying people 75 years and younger with AD, she found

that those who had worked in occupations with higher EMF exposures were five times more likely to develop AD. [12]

- In 2007, Ana Garcia of the University of Valencia, Spain, published a meta-analysis of the studies done on occupational links to AD. She reported that the combined data from 14 different occupational studies showing that being exposed to EMFs on the job doubled the risk of developing AD.[13]

The research on the negative impact from cell phones and WI-FI on brains and nervous system functions is even more frightening. The results leave little doubt that the wide spread use of WI-FI and cell phones is causing an acceleration of Alzheimer's in an aging population.

> The main contribution to the increased mortality in nervous system related diseases was deaths due to increasing mortality in Alzheimer's disease (AD). The correlation between mobile phone average output power and mortality has increased the last few years and is today significant.... "The mortality in Alzheimer's disease appears to be associated with mobile phone output power. The mortality is increasing fast and is expected to increase substantially within the next 10 years.[12]

The many health risks for the brain associated with cell phone and WI-FI are real and should be taken seriously. Here are quotes from several researchers and organizations concerning these health risks.

> Any possible health effects of the ELF-EMFs would be of concern because powerlines and electrical devices are present everywhere is modern life, and people are constantly encountering these fields, both in their homes and in certain workplaces. Also, the presence of ELF-EMFs in homes means that children are exposed. Even if ELF-EMFs were to increase an individual's risk of disease only slightly, widespread exposure to ELF-EMFs could translate to meaningful increased risks at the population level.
> National Cancer Institute.[13]

Cells in the body react to EMFs as potentially harmful, just like other environmental toxins including heavy metals and toxic chemicals. The DNA in living cells recognizes electromagnetic fields at very low levels of exposure and produces a biochemical stress of response.
Dr. Reba Goodman, PhD, professor emeritus, clinical pathology, Columbia University.[14]

Children are more vulnerable to RF/MW radiation because of the susceptibility of their developing nervous systems. RF/MW penetration is greater relative to head size in children, who have a greater absorption of RF/MW energy in the tissues of the head at W-Fi frequencies. Such greater absorption results because children's heads are thinner, their brains are smaller, and their brain tissue is more conductive than those of adults since it has a higher water content and concentrations.
Dr. David O. Carpenter, MD, director of the Institute for Health and the Environment at the University at Albany and co-editor of the *Biointiative Report*.[15, 16]

Radio frequency radiation and other forms of the electromagnetic pollution are harmful at orders of magnitude well below existing guidelines. Science is one of the tools society uses to decide health policy. In the case of telecommunications equipment, such as cell phones, wireless networks, cell phone antennas, PDAs, and portable phones, the science is being ignored. Current guidelines urgently need to be re-examined by government and reduced to reflect the state of the science. There is an emerging public health crisis at hand and time is of the essence. – Dr. Magda Havas, PhD, associate professor, environment and resource studies, Trent University.[17]

Exposure to radio-frequency, or RF, radiation is a major risk of cellphone use. Manufacturers have a legal duty to provide warnings that are clear and conspicuous when products raise health and safety concerns. But, typically, RF safety

instructions are buried in user manuals with tiny print, hidden within smartphones, or made available on the internet.
Dr. Joel Moskowitz, PhD, director of the Center for Family and Community Health, University of California, Berkley.[18]

There are many examples of the failure to use the precautionary principle in the past, which have resulted in serious and often irreversible damage to health and environments. Appropriate, precautionary and proportionate actions taken now to avoid plausible and potentially serious threats to health from EMF are likely to be seen as prudent and wise from future perspectives.
Jacqueline Mc Glade, chief scientist, United Nations Environment Program.[19]

I do think that the amount of radiation exposure we get these days is exponentially higher than we did 15-20 years ago. So anything you can do to limit your exposure to radiation is a good idea. But I don't think you need to give up these products. I try not to put the laptop directly on my lap, I try not to put the cell phone in my ear.
Dr. Sanjay Gupta, MD, CNN chief medical correspondent.[20]

The biggest problem we have is that we know most environmental factors take several decades of exposure before we really see the consequences.
Dr. Keith Black, chairman of neurology at Cedars- Sinai Medical Center, Los Angeles.[21]

Really at the heart of my concern is that we shouldn't wait for a definitive study to come out, but err on the side of being safe rather than sorry later.
Dr. Ronald B. Herberman, University of Pittsburg Cancer Institute.[22]

EMFs, potential stressors causing inflammation, belong in the category of environmental toxins along with heavy metals like mercury and aluminum and pesticides like glyphosate. Although this chapter is about the aging brain—dementia/Alzheimer's disease, you also need to be aware of the dangers to children as it relates to the current epidemic of learning and behavioral problems associated with ADHD and autism spectrum disorders. EMFs and other environmental toxins found in air, water, and food sources are adversely affecting developing fetuses in the womb and in early formative years.[23]

The gaps in research raise additional concerns for specific individuals. Here is a possible worst-case scenario. The individual has had a concussion with loss of consciousness and has the APOE4 gene variant (now at increased 10x risk), works in an occupation that has high EMF exposure (another 4x risk), doesn't get adequate omega3 fatty acids (2x risk), and has low thyroid function (2x risk), raising this individual's risk160x for developing Alzheimer's. As a health practitioner, I don't know the relative risk of having all these factors with certainly because no one has done this type of study. I do know that the more risk factors the more likely a person is to have AD. And I can change these risk factors by supplementing with adequate niacin and having the person get regular exercise to help negate the APOE4 gene. I can test for fatty acids and hypothyroid function and supplement accordingly. The individual can reduce the EMF exposure. While s/he cannot go back in time and prevent the concussion, the individual can effectively treat the brain and restore circulation and mitochondrial energy to the brain with the infra-red light harness and stimulate more healing gamma waves with the BrainTap.

Being better informed allows me and the public to become more preventative because there will never be a magic drug invented that is going to turn around a brain that has lost 80-90 % of the functioning neurons in a specific area. Here are some things you can do to minimize your exposure to EMFs.

1. Use Ethernet cables to hardwire networks instead of using over-the-air transmissions.
2. Place the router at least ten feet or more where people are active, place in the least active areas.
3. Do not put wireless routers near bedrooms.
4. For children, avoid using WI-FI in schools, nurseries, day care centers, and playrooms.
5. Turn your Wi-Fi off at night. You don't need Wi-Fi on while you sleep—having it on can actually interfere with your

sleep. There are many devices you can install in your home to make this process easy.

6. Keep your phone on airplane mode as much as possible.
7. Keep your phone off your body when you're not using it.
8. Stay away from Bluetooth devices, and opt for wired headphones instead.
9. Put technology away two hours before bed if you can. Not only are the EMFs harmful but blue light from your computer and phone screen after dark reduce melatonin levels, your most powerful endogenous anti-oxidant. Consider reading the Bible, positive self-help books, or a humorous book or magazine, watching a comedy, meditating, taking a hot bath or sauna, doing some yoga, or doing a BrainTap session.

Reference List

1. California Development of Public Health. *How to reduce exposure to radiofrequency energy from cell phones.* https://www.cdph.ca.gov/Programs/CCDPHP/DEODC/EHIB /CDPH%20Document%20Library/Cell-Phone-Guidance.pdf. Accessed Apr 13, 2018.
2. Rodriguez M, Petitclerc D, Burchard JF, Nguyen DH, Block E. Blood melatonin and prolactin concentrations in dairy cows exposed to 60 Hz electric and magnetic fields during 8 hour photoperiods. *BioElectroMagnetics*:16 September 2004.
3. Burchard JF, Nguyen DH, Rodriguez M. Plasma concentrations of thyroxine in dairy cows exposed to 60 Hz electric and magnetic fields. *BioElectroMagnetics*: 24 May 2006.
4. Gorpinchenko I, Nikitin O, Banyra O, Shulyak A. The influence of direct mobile phone radiation on sperm quality. *Cent European J Urol* 2014; 67(1): 65-71. doi: 10.5173/ceju.2014.01.art14.
5. Qui C, Fratiglioni L, Karp A, Winblad B, Bellander T. Occupational Exposure to Electromagnetic Fields and Risk of Alzheimer's. *Epidemology*: November 2004; 15(6):687-94.
6. Hakansson N, Gustavsson P, Johansen C, Floderus B. Neurodegenerative Diseases in Welders and other Workers

Exposed to high Levels of Magnetic Fields. *Epidemiology:* July 2003;14(4)420-426.

7. DeBaun DT, DeBaun RP. *Radiation Nation.* Venice, FL: Icaro Publishing. 2017.

8. Tompkins P, Bird C. *The Secret Life of Plants.* New York: Harper & Row, 1989.

9. The National Academics of Sciences Engineering Medicine. *Assessment of the Possible Health Effects of Groundwave Emergency Network.* Washington, DC: The National Academies Press, 1993.

10. Davanipour Z, Tseng C-C, Lee P-J, Sorbel E. A case-control study of occupational magnetic field exposure and Alzheimer's disease: results from the California Alzheimer's Disease Diagnosis and Treatment Centers. *MC Neurology* 2007 June 9;7:13.

11. Sobel E, Davanipour Z, Sulkava R et al. Occupations with Exposure to Electromagnetic Field: A Possible Risk Factor for Alzheimer's Disease. *American Journal of Epidemiology* 1995 Sep 1; 142(5): 515-524.

12. Sobel E, Dunn Z, Davanipour Z, Qian Z, Chui HC. Elevated risk of Alzheimer's disease among workers with likely electromagnetic field exposure. *Neurology* Dec 01, 1996; 47(6).

13. National Cancer Institute. Magnetic field exposure and cancer. *Fact Sheet.* https://www.hydroone.com/poweroutagesandsafety_/corporat ehealthandsafety_/EMFs/Magnetic_Field_Exposure_and_Ca ncer.pdf. Accessed Apr 14, 2018.

14. Feychting M, Jonsson F, Pedersen N, Ahlbom A. Occupational Magnetic Field Exposure and Neurodegenerative Disease. *Epidemiology* July 2003; 4(14): 413-419.

15. Mottus, K. *Health effect dangers of WiFi in schools—David Carpenter.* June 3, 2014. http://www.smartvoter.org/2014/06/03/ca/state/vote/mottus_ k/paper2.html. Accessed Apr 14, 2018.

16. Carpenter, DM, Sage C. *Bioinitiative Report 2012.* http://www.bioinitiative.org/. Accessed Apr 14, 2018.

17. Flynn A. *Dear broadband technologies opportunities programs.* Apr 6, 2009. http://www.ntia.doc.gov/broadbandgrants/form.cfm. Accessed Apr 14, 2018.
18. Moskowitz J. *Electromagnetic Radiation Safety.* https://ecfsapi.fcc.gov/file/60002030879.pdf. Accessed Apr 14, 2018.
19. McGlade J. *III. Statement on mobile phones by executive director of European Environment Agency.* http://www.sehn.org/rpr187.html#T3. Accessed Apr 14, 2018.
20. DefenderShield. *What experts say about EMF radiation and our health.* https://www.defendershield.com/learn/experts/. Accessed Apr 14, 2018.
21. Dellorto D. WHO: cell phone use can increase possible cancer risk. *CNN* 2011 May 31. http://edition.cnn.com/2011/HEALTH/05/31/who.cell.phones/index.html. Accessed Apr 14, 2018.
22. Pitt's cancer institute warns staff about possible cell phone use. *Daily News* 2008 Jul 23. http://www.nydailynews.com/life-style/health/pitt-cancer-institute-warns-staff-cell-phone-risks-article-1.351923. Accessed Apr 14, 2018.
23. Bellini CV, Pinto I. Fetal and neonatal effects of EMF. In D M Carpenter & C Sage (eds.) *Bioinitiative Report 2012.* http://www.bioinitiative.org/. Accessed Apr 14, 2018.

Conclusion and Recommendations

Despite accumulating evidence of the harmful effects of environmental toxins, there has been limited efforts to curb exposure for the majority of people. In 1976, the Toxic Substances Control Act (TSCA) was passed. This was a very weak law particularly in terms of enforcement. That was 40 years ago and it was never updated until 2000. At that time, 62,000 different chemicals were grandfathered in and presumed safe. The law did not require any safety study to be done before a chemical was allowed on the market. The FDA approved 90% of all new chemicals within 3 weeks with only five chemicals having been restricted. The law was so weak that when the Bush administration tried to ban asbestos the manufacturers challenged it in court and won. This law was strengthened during the Obama administration.[1]

Other laws have been more effective. In 1972, when lead was removed from gasoline, blood levels for lead in the average U.S. citizen were 100 ppb. Today, the average levels are down to 4 ppb.[2] Despite this one change and the elimination of lead in paint, lead poisoning continues to be in the news, especially in terms of water quality.[3] You might also be surprised to discover how many older Americans still have significant toxic lead levels in their bodies. The last time I did a self-evaluation on myself, both lead and mercury levels were still elevated.

While PCBs were introduced in the 1930s, they were not evaluated until the 1970s. In 1973, PCB level averaged 15 ppb. In 1976, PCBs were banned and average levels had dropped to 1.24 ppb by 1991. Even today, certain individuals have significantly higher levels.[4] The pesticide DDT has been used since 1938. In 1972, average levels in humans were 8,000 ppb. When DDT was banned that same year, levels decreased to 5145 ppb by 1974, to 2340 ppb by 1986, and to 260 ppb by 1999.[5] Given this ban, it is surprising that 97% of those living in the U.S. still have detectable levels of DDT in their bloodstream.[6] As recently as 2004, blood in the umbilical cord of ten newborn babies still contained PCBs and DDT.[7]

In 2008, the Kid-Safe Chemical Act (KSCA) was passed and updated versions were passed in 2010, 2012, and 2013. This act forced a company to prove a chemical was safe before they brought it to market. The act assumed that any chemical was potentially hazardous until proven otherwise and priority was given to those chemicals found in the umbilical cord in the 2004 Ten Americans Study[7] because they can pass on to the brain.[8] Despite this progress. more needs to be done. Unfortunately, the pharmaceutical and industrial chemical industries have plenty of money to sponsor and publish questionable and biased research to demonstrate their products are safe even when they are not. More unbiased independent research from organizations like the Environment Working Group (EWG) is needed to help ensure our safety.

Reference List

1. McCarthy G. TSCA reform: a bipartisan milestone to protect our health from dangerous chemicals. *The EPA Blog,* June 22, 2016. https://blog.epa.gov/blog/2016/06/tsca-reform-a-bipartisan-milestone-to-protect-our-health-from-dangerous-chemicals/. Accessed Mar 24, 2018.
2. Greenfield N. *Lead by the numbers.* Feb 18, 2016. https://www.nrdc.org/onearth/lead-numbers. Accessed Mar 25, 2018.
3. Pupovac J. Where lead lurks and why even small amounts matter. *Shots: health news from NPR.* Aug 12, 2016. https://www.npr.org/sections/health-shots/2016/08/12/483079525/where-lead-lurks-and-why-even-small-amounts-matter. Accessed Mar 25, 2018.
4. Environmental Protection Agency. *Review of PCB levels in the environment.* 1976. https://nepis.epa.gov/Exe/ZyNET.exe/2000I3HT.TXT?ZyActionD=ZyDocument&Client=EPA&Index=1976+Thru+1980&Docs=&Query=&Time=&EndTime=&SearchMethod=1&TocRestrict=n&Toc=&TocEntry=&QField=&QFieldYear=&QFieldMonth=&QFieldDay=&IntQFieldOp=0&ExtQFieldOp=0&XmlQuery=&File=D%3A%5Czyfiles%5CIndex%20Data%5C76thru80%5CTxt%5C00000002%5C2000I3HT.txt&User=ANONYMOUS&Password=anonymous&SortMethod=h%7C-&MaximumDocuments=1&FuzzyDegree=0&ImageQuality=r75g8/r75g8/x150y150g16/i425&Display=hpfr&DefSeekPag

e=x&SearchBack=ZyActionL&Back=ZyActionS&BackDesc
=Results%20page&MaximumPages=1&ZyEntry=1&SeekPa
ge=x&ZyPURL. Accessed Mar 24, 2018.

5. Environmental Working Group. *10 Americans.* [videotape]. Washington, DC: EWG; 2012.
6. Environmental Working Group. *10 Americans.* [videotape]. Washington, DC: EWG; 2012.
7. Environmental Working Group. *Body burden: the pollution in newborns.* July 14, 2005. https://www.ewg.org/research/body-burden-pollution-newborn. Accessed Mar 25, 2018.
8. Duvall M, Lewis C, Wyatt A. *The Kid-Safe Chemicals Act: a potential change to the Toxic Substances Control Act.* Jan 2009. http://www.bdlaw.com/assets/htmldocuments/KID-SAFE%20CHEMICALS%20ACT%20ANALYSIS.pdf. Accessed Mar 25, 2018.

Recommendations

There are some things that you can do to reduce toxic environmental exposure. To protect yourself and your family, I recommend some action steps to help give you peace of mind protection at the home and office. Improvement of the quality of your air and water are foundational to a healthier life.

1. Support local and national environment watchdog groups. They have you, your children, and grandchildren's best interest at heart.

2. Write and talk to your senators and congressmen. Be a label reader. Use environmental friendly, green products.

3. Become pro-active in the community and politically to protect your environment.

4. Stop drinking bottled water. Almost 50% contain tap water and all contain micro-plastics that are toxic and accumulate in your body.

5. Use the Multipure™ solid carbon block filter to remove as many environmental toxins out as possible. (These are available from this website: www.healthrestoration.solutions. See Peace of Mind Protection Package.)

6. Electrically reduce the purified water from the Multipure™ with the Living Water system to make anti-oxidant water to help

---

151

reduce ROS (reactive oxygen species) in the body. (These are available from this website: www.drkellymiller.com. See Peace of Mind Protection Package.)

7. Drink your water from stainless steel or glass-lined containers.

8. Reduce transdermal introduction of petrochemicals by using the Multipure™ house protection and Laundry Pure that cleans clothes in cold water without laundry detergents and fabric softeners. (These are available from this website: www.drkellymiller.com. See Peace of Mind Protection Package.)

9. Reduce reoccurring airborne toxins from indoor air pollution by using the NASA approved air filtration Active Pure system at your home and office. (These are available from this website: www.drkellymiller.com. See "Peace of Mind" Protection Package.)

10. Reduce/eliminate GMO foods from your diet. Eat organic foods as often as possible.

11. Reduce exposure to EMFs as outlined in that chapter.

Supplementation Recommendations
1. Increase supplementation of anti-oxidants, such as glutathione, catalase, and super-oxide dismutase.
2. Increase supplementation of methylated B vitamins.
3. Increase supplementation of D3/K2.
4. Increase supplementation of healthy 3-6-9 fatty acids.
5. Take probiotics.

Recommended Testing
1. Do the MRT evaluation to determine food/chemical allergy/sensitivity and eliminate these. (Kits available from this website: www.drkellymiller.com.)
2. Do thyroflex testing for your thyroid and saliva hormone testing for your sex hormones to evaluate if your endocrine system is functioning optimally. (Kits available from this website: www.drkellymiller.com.)
3. Do organic acid/environmental testing to determine levels of excess toxins and what nutrients you need to eliminate these. (Kits available from this website: www.drkellymiller.com.)

4. Do micronutrient testing to determine deficiency/adequacy of key nutrients that are involved in detoxification/anti-oxidation and mitochondrial energy. (Kits available from this website: www.drkellymiller.com.)
5. Go to www.drkellymiller.com to get a customized personalized nutraceutical support program.

Appendix

Case History #1

AP was a 48-year-old male who was referred to me by his treating chiropractor in Lincoln, Nebraska. His chief complaints were brain fog, digestive dysfunction, low energy, and poor sleep. AP had quite a detailed journaled health history he shared with me. Of significance was a history of multiple vaccinations in Peru in the year 2000. He traveled there on two occasions, staying there for approximately one month each visit. AP related most of his symptomatology began or magnified during this time period.

AP like many of my patients had seen several other physicians prior to his consultation with me in an attempt to ameliorate his numerous symptoms. In addition, he spent a great deal of time on the internet searching for solutions. AP was taking multiple different nutraceuticals in an attempt to correct his conditions. Several years prior to this consultation with me, he had consulted with a physician in St. Louis who ordered GI testing. He also consulted another physician who had ordered IgG food testing and hair analysis for heavy metals. In addition, he had seen a physician who ordered an extensive thyroid panel, including TPOab. He had been told that he had antibodies, but had not been given any specific plan to address the problem. The presence of the TPOab is significant for a diagnosis of Hashimoto's disease, an auto-immune condition causing hypothyroidism.

I asked AP to fill out some questionnaires prior to our consultation: a system survey form, a thyroflex questionnaire to help identify thyroid, adrenal, and melatonin issues, and a Braverman questionnaire. The system survey questionnaire evaluates autonomic nervous system function: sympathetic (fight/flight) and parasympathetic (digestion and healing), blood sugar regulation, liver, gallbladder function, cardiovascular function, and the endocrine function of the adrenals, thyroid, and pituitary. The thyroflex questionnaire asked additional questions related to thyroid, adrenal, and sleep function. The Braverman questionnaires are designed to help determine the dominant neurotransmitter of the brain: dopamine, acetylcholine, GABA, or serotonin, and any deficiency levels of these four neurotransmitters. AP had several complaints related to brain function, such as anxiety, memory dysfunction, sleep issues. The system survey indicated that the vast majority of symptoms were related to four areas: 1. digestive dysfunction, 2. hormone dysfunction, 3. liver, biliary (gallbladder) dysfunction, and 4. blood sugar dysregulation. His thyroflex questionnaire indicated hypofunction of the thyroid and adrenals and the need for melatonin and 5 HTP.

My recommendations for testing consisted of a comprehensive stool analysis with parasitology, blood spot thyroid panel, saliva sex hormone panel, micronutrients panel, organic acid panel, GPL-Tox Non-Metal Environmental panel, and glyphosate panel. These tests gave me the best information to evaluate AP's signs and symptoms. When consulting with patient, I look to the 9 variables of health and longevity—genetic variants, environmental toxins, trauma, what they eat, what they drink, how they exercise, how they rest, how/what they breathe, and what they think—as the potential causative factors in their dysfunction. These 9 potential stressors cause the 7 sequela of stress: autonomic nervous system imbalance, hormone imbalance/deficiencies, micronutrient deficiencies, sticky blood/platelets, damage to the glycocalyx/endothelium of the blood vessels, and loss of Secretory IgA/leaky gut/microbiome change, and mitochondrial DNA changes.

AP's test results revealed the following: His TSH (thyroid-stimulating hormone) was 10.0 uU/mL. Normal reference range at this lab was 0.5-3.0 uU/mL. His TPO antibodies were positive at 89 IU/mL—normal is < 1 IU/ml, so AP had Hashimoto's hypothyroid, an autoimmune hypothyroid condition. His free T4, free T3 levels were within reference range. However, I must tell you that many people have a normal TSH that have Hashimoto's. TPO is rarely checked by the most physicians.

The Braverman questionnaire indicated AP demonstrated dopamine dominant neurotransmitter characteristics with severe deficiencies of GABA and serotonin. Dopamine is a stimulatory neurotransmitter while GABA and serotonin are inhibitory neurotransmitters. In essence, as far as AP's brain function was concerned, the accelerator was on the floorboard and the brakes were not working. This was contributing to or causing his anxiousness, insomnia and intermittent mental fog. His hypothyroid condition was negatively influencing his neurotransmitters.

Hypothyroidism is epidemic in this country affecting approximately 80% of the adult population, of which the vast majority are undiagnosed. The reasons for the hypothyroidism epidemic are multiple. I go into these in detail in my book, *13 Secrets to Optimal Aging: How Your Hormone System Can Help You Achieve Qualitative Health and Longevity.*

New information from a 100,000-patient database tested with an FDA cleared diagnostic device called the thyroflex confirms these statistics. Of these 100,000 people evaluated, 80 % percent demonstrated hypothyroidism. One in 5 or 20% of those affected had Hashimoto's disease. Autoimmune disorders are often multiple in individuals. If you have been diagnosed with an autoimmune disorder, such as rheumatoid arthritis, scleroderma, multiple sclerosis, lupus, or Sjorden's syndrome, you may also have Hashimoto's thyroiditis.

Four specific environmental toxins of heavy body burden identified from the GPL-Tox panel were also contributing to AP's negative symptoms. The first was a marker for a gasoline additive that is used to increase octane ratings in gasoline. Exposure to this compound is through inhalation, skin exposure to gasoline, its vapors, or exhaust fumes, or ground water. Since AP had no history of working in or around gasoline, I presumed it originated from his water intake. I recommended a Multipure™ solid carbon filter to remove this toxin from his drinking water. This chemical like many others is not monitored by the EPA or municipalities.

The second chemical detected was perchlorate that was found in high concentrations, in the 95th percentile. This means AP tested for concentrations levels that are higher than 95% of thousands of others tested. This chemical is used in the production of rocket fuel, missiles, fireworks, flares, explosives, and bleach. Studies show it is often found in drinking water. Perchlorate can disrupt the thyroid's ability to make hormones. The EPA lists perchlorate as a likely human carcinogen. Reverse osmosis and Multipure™ systems can remove this toxin from the drinking water. Because the Aquaperform Multipure™ system can remove more contaminants than reverse osmosis, I recommend this to my patients.

The third toxin found in AP above the 95th percentile was DMP, organophosphates. It is one of the most toxic groups of substances in the world and found primarily in pesticide formulations. Organophosphates can lead to overstimulation of neurons or muscles, resulting in excessive salivation, abnormal behavior, diarrhea, urinary incontinence, vomiting, tremors, muscle paralysis, and even death. High exposure levels have been associated with attention deficit, memory impairment, and pervasive developmental disorders. Exposure has also been linked to violent behavior, depression, and suicide and may have a role in the onset of Gulf War syndrome. Organophosphate exposure can be reduced by eating organic foods, avoiding using pesticides in house or garden, avoiding living near agricultural areas or golf courses, and staying indoors if insecticides are being sprayed. Lice shampoo, pet flea collars, and flea spray are also major sources of organophosphates. Ground water is a source. Remove sources of exposure if possible. Elimination of organophosphates can be accelerated by sauna treatment. These compounds are another reason for using Mulitpure™.

One other toxin found in gasoline was found to be at the 50th percentile. Because ETBE/MTBE has an excretion half-life of 10-28 hours, his score suggests he was getting routine exposure to a bad water supply as he had no exposure to gasoline vapors a few days prior to testing. Infrared sauna increases the excretion as well as reduced glutathione and N-acetylcysteine (NAC). These nutrients were put in his personalized nutritional recommendations. Because stopping the reoccurring poisoning was a must, this is another reason I recommended the Multipure™ solid carbon block water filter.

AP also exhibited decreased levels of testosterone, DHEA, and cortisol and elevated levels of estrone and estradiol. These are common findings in the aging male, especially after age 50. In AP's case, he was only 48. Seeing these problems in younger men is a modern trend as I have seen hormone problems with men in their twenties. DHEA and cortisol are produced by the adrenal cortex. Low levels indicate hypofunction of the adrenals or adrenal fatigue. In addition, lower levels of DHEA and cortisol cause a decrease in the amount of Secretory IgA, the mucous membrane that protects the digestive system, allowing hyper permeability, aka leaky gut. Although the Secretory IgA was within reference range in comprehensive GI panel, it was in the lowest quintile (20%).

Other data from his comprehensive stool panel revealed he had no significant growth of the Bifidobacterium species. This is one of the most common and normally abundant bacteria in the colon. Elevated levels of lysozyme were found. Lysozyme is an enzyme secreted at the site of inflammation in the GI tract, and elevated levels have been identified in IBD patients. White Blood Cells (WBC) and mucous in the stool can occur with bacterial and parasitic infections, with mucosal irritation, and inflammatory bowel diseases, such as Crohn's disease or ulcerative colitis. High levels of yeast, Geotrichim spp, and Rhodororula mucilagenosa, were found. Luckily, these had very high sensitivity to grapeseed extract. The challenge for consumers with using grapeseed extract is finding one that is not loaded with pesticides.

The food/chemical allergy/sensitivity test called MRT (mediator release test) revealed a moderate reactivity to the chemicals phenylethylalanine, FD&C Blue #1, FD&C Red #4, saccharine, polysorbate 80, and a severe reactivity to FD&C #40. These inflammatory reactions are fairly common, and I caution parents to read the labels of all foods they and their children consume. Additionally, AP exhibited a severe reactivity to cow's milk and moderate reactivity to cayenne pepper, dill, ginger, garlic, avocado, grape, sweet potato, beet, spinach, kamut, barley, corn, scallop, cola, coffee, tea, soybean, peanut, and almond. Many of these—ginger, garlic, grape, sweet potato, beet, spinach, and almonds—are normally considered healthy foods. In the case of AP these were causing him inflammation. After 60 days, he was allowed to rotate among these foods a couple times a week. AP had well over 100 different foods he could choose from that did not cause high inflammation. These were his grocery list for the next 60 days. Positive results are usually seen within two weeks of eliminating the reactive (inflammatory) foods.

Spectracell's micronutrients test results demonstrated a severe deficiency of L-serine, an amino acid important in the myelin sheath and brain integrity, and in Vitamin B1, thiamine. Borderline deficiencies in other B vitamins—B3 (niacin), B6, pantothenate, folate, and B12, glutathione glutamine, oleic acid (found in olive oil), and calcium were found. Overall. he was also found to be borderline deficient in his antioxidant capacity. Replenishing glutathione levels took care of the anti-oxidant capacity. Consequently, I recommended nutritional repletion of these nutrients.

The Organic Acids Test revealed abnormalities for 8 different markers related to yeast/fungal overgrowth in the gastrointestinal tract. Natural antifungal products as well as 100 million CFU probiotics were recommended. A detected high hippuric acid marker indicated bacterial overgrowth. The recommended probiotic handled this condition as well.

The presence of high lactic and pyruvic acid markers indicated bacterial overgrowth or a mitochondrial deficiency of pantothenic acid, FAD derived from riboflavin, or thiamine. I recommended B vitamins for these conditions. I also recommended supplementation of riboflavin, COQ10, NAD (nicotinamide-adenine dinucleotide, a coenzyme that is involved in many biochemi cal oxidation-reductions), l-carnitine, nicotinamide, biotin, and Vitamin E to benefit the mitochondrial energy production: The presence of high succinic and fumaric acid markers indicated mitochondrial energy dysfunction.

Low levels of HVA and VMA markers were present, which are highly suggestive of low levels of phenylalanine and tyrosine, amino acids. Supplementation indicated the co-factors of magnesium, B6 (pyridoxine), and biopterin, a coenzyme that's used to make several important neurotransmitters in the body. The low 5-HIAA marker indicated the lower production neurotransmitter serotonin. This was also indicated by the Braverman questionnaire. Supplementation of 5-HTP (5-hydroxytrytophan) is usually beneficial for this condition. Other markers indicated increased metabolic utilization of fatty acids. These markers may be associated with diabetes, fasting, or a ketogenic diet, which is so popular now. However, it usually means there is a deficiency of carnitine, which is a limiting factor in being able to use fatty acids for mitochondrial energy. AP also had markers that indicated a need for B6 and other methylated B vitamins, such as riboflavin, folate, B12, and glutathione.

In summary, AP had several concomitant conditions that needed to be addressed. They were the following.

1. Autonomic nervous system imbalance (anxiety/sleep disturbance/digestion)
2. Hypothyroid (Hashimoto's)
3. Multiple sex hormone imbalances/deficiencies
4. Multiple micronutrient deficiencies
5. Heavy body burden of multiple environmental toxins

6. Multiple food/chemical allergies/sensitivities
7. Leaky gut
8. Microbiome imbalance with yeast/pathological bacteria overgrowth
9. Neurotransmitter imbalance/deficiencies (anxiety)
10. Mitochondrial energy problems

My approach to handling these problems is two-fold. I must first stop the poisoning of the body that is causing chronic inflammation and overwhelming the detoxification and immune systems. The first thing I do is to ensure a pure water source by installing an Aquaperform Multipure™ solid carbon filter for all drinking water. The second is to have the patient stop eating all reactive foods for 60 days. This gives relief for leaky gut, microbiome, hormone system, and neurotransmitters. The auto-immune response is due to an over-reaction of the immune system most probably due to a food/chemical allergy/sensitivity going through the leaky gut. This could be from gluten or wheat gliadins (proteins), casein (milk protein), or others. The chronic inflammation causes the leaky gut and microbiome imbalance. The microbiome influences the neurotransmitters as they are responsible for 90 % of the production. Elimination of reactive foods/chemical stops the inflammatory process, which stops the leaky gut and microbiome imbalances. It has been my experience that this often reduces the number of TPO antibodies of Hashimoto's as well. One of the reasons many patients are not able to get well is because they do not stop the poisons coming into their bodies.

The second step I use is to shore up the many deficiencies that showed up on through testing. Supplementation recommendations were made to kill the yeast/bacteria overgrowth and to re-implant an abundance of diverse, good bacteria. It should be noted that if you try a large dose of probiotics and you get increased bloating and gas that you may have what is known as SIBO (small intestine bacteria overgrowth). This can be tested for through an inhalation test. Supplementation recommendations were made for thyroid and adrenal support and bio-identical hormone replacement. The hormones are anti-oxidant and anti-inflammatory and positively influence the neurotransmitters. Supplementation was

161

also made for the numerous nutrients lacking through the Spectracell's Micronutrient Test, Organic Acid Test, and the GPL-Tox Non-Metal Chemical Test. The vast majority of the nutrients were made in a customized formula through IDlife. I find that I can replenish 80-90% of the nutrients patients need through this methodology. Idlife^{TM} is a HIPPA compliant platform that has a patented process of replacing nutrient deficiencies caused by medications. It also keeps nutrients out or limits the dosing of a nutrient that may be contra-indicated by a medication specific or condition. There are over 300 condition-specific recommendations. The patient feels out a detailed questionnaire on-line that takes into account genetics, allergies, family history, personal history, and lifestyle. There are approximately 5,500 variables resulting in a potential 1.7 million different nutritional recommendations. I find it quite accurate in predicting what an individual needs. The platform allows me the freedom to add other nutrients as well.

In the particular case of AP, many of his symptoms improved just within two weeks of avoiding the reactive foods. Within two months he was 80 % better. He was still having some intermittent bloating and mental fog that was relieved when we added some additional grapefruit extract to help with his candida. Long-term goals were to help him manage his Hashimoto's disease. Hashimoto's like other auto-immune diseases can be managed by finding and eliminating the inflammatory triggers. Auto-immune disease is like a fire. It starts as a tiny ember, but unmanaged turns into a roaring fire. The fuel for the fire can be gluten, wheat gliadins (proteins), casein, mercury, arsenic, fluoride, bromide, or some other food(s) and/or chemical(s).

Case History #2

NB was a 60-year-old female physician who was slender, a vegetarian who ate only organic food, and exercised regularly. She was diagnosed with breast cancer and had a double mastectomy with chemotherapy in the past year prior to my consultation with her. Her energy was low, and she did not have much initiative or endurance. NB wanted to know how to be as healthy as she could be at this point. I listened to her history, reviewed prior test results, told her about the approach I planned to take based upon my analysis and why she was experiencing the loss of initiative and endurance. NB had some genetic testing done that indicated she had the BRAC gene variant, which increased her risk for breast and uterine cancer. It should be kept in mind that even the BRAC gene is actionable and can be positively influenced by adequate methylation of B Vitamins, Vitamin D, and anti-oxidants like glutathione. NB had elected a voluntary removal of her uterus prior to the time of the consultation.

Based on her history and information obtained from the intake forms, I determined it necessary to evaluate her thyroid function via the thyroflex and blood spot testing, sex hormones through salivary testing, Organic Acid Test, GPL-Tox Non-Metal Chemical Profile, Glyphosate Test through urinalysis, the Micronutrient Test, and MRT (Mediator Release Test) for food/chemical allergy/sensitivity through a blood draw. These were done in order to ascertain the underlying potential stressors in her environment and what nutritional/hormonal deficiencies she currently had. Because the hormones are the first line of defense and so many different environmental toxins adversely impact the hormones, I wanted to evaluate how her endocrine system—the thyroid, adrenals, and gonads (ovaries)—was functioning.

I conducted a thyroflex test in the office to evaluate her intracellular T3 levels. The thyroflex test is a non-invasive FDA cleared device that determines intracellular T3 levels with a 98.5% accuracy through brachioradialis reflexometry. Ideal readings of reflex speed for a person with optimum thyroid function are from 50-100 milliseconds. Satisfactory or marginal readings are from 100-120 milliseconds. NB's readings were at 189 milliseconds, indicative of hypothyroid function. Her TSH, free T4, free T3 levels were within reference range like so many other undiagnosed hypothyroid patients. However, her average basal body temperature over 5 mornings was 97.4 degrees, another indicator of hypothyroid function. Most important she had multiple symptoms of hypothyroidism that were confirmed by the thyroflex test results. I suspect that these discrepancies in blood testing and symptoms are due to a combination of the reference ranges being used that had been normed on a sick population, the blood tests are less accurate than previously believed, and widespread thyroid receptor resistance.

A saliva hormone test was also ordered to monitor her sex hormones: progesterone, estrone, estradiol, estriol, testosterone, DHEA, and cortisol. Saliva readings were taken 5 times throughout the day and revealed low levels of progesterone, an important hormone in reducing risk for breast cancer, low cortisol level both morning and night, low levels of testosterone, and extremely low level of DHEA. Estrone levels were slightly elevated. This is significant because it is the estrone metabolites of 16-alpha-hydroxyestrone and 4-hydroxyestrone that are potentially carcinogenic. Low progesterone and elevated estrone levels are a bad combination for someone trying to avoid breast, uterine, or ovarian cancer. Testosterone, DHEA, and cortisol are all produced by the adrenal cortex area. If they were low, there is adrenal hypofunction or fatigue. Low DHEA and cortisol in combination causes a loss of Secretory IgA, the mucosal layer in the gastrointestinal tract to protect against microorganisms. This in turn causes hyperpermability, aka leaky gut, in an individual.

A large panel of 1000 SNPs (Single Nucleotide Polymorphism) was ordered to determine if there were other gene variants in addition to the BRAC gene that could put her at risk for cancers, especially estrogen-related cancers. An SNP is the most common type of gene variant. NB had 35 different gene variants related to DNA methylation, which were involved directly or indirectly to estrogen detoxification, that necessitated a reduced form of folate and a significantly greater amount of methylated B vitamins like riboflavin, B6, and B12. She also had two gene variants for COMT (catechol-O-methyltransferase), an enzyme that is critical for proper estrogen detoxification. These gene variants necessitated 300-400% greater need for methylated B vitamins. NB also had VDR (Vitamin D receptor) gene variants. Studies show that adequate Vitamin D and calcium can reduce the risk of breast cancer by 70 %. Not knowing this and consequently not supplementing with increased Vitamin D levels had increased her breast cancer risk and greatly contributed to her development of osteoporosis. She also had several SNPs that increased her risk for neurological disorders and gluten sensitivity. She did not have the APOE4 gene variant that increases the risk for Alzheimer's. NB will always need to take significantly increased doses of methylated B vitamins and Vitamin D to compensate for these gene variants.

A food/chemical allergy/sensitivity test was ordered through Oxford labs. The MRT (Mediator Release Test) revealed multiple foods/chemicals that were reactive and causing an inflammatory reaction to sodium sulfite, millet, and wheat and moderate reactivity to FD &C green dye, yogurt, American cheese, olives, plums, soybeans, sweet potatoes, white potatoes, mushrooms, lettuce, zucchini, baker's yeast, crab, salmon, and sole. Because of the number and variety of foods and chemicals, it would have been virtually impossible to figure this out on her own with an elimination-type diet.

It is essential that these reactive foods be avoided for a period of time to reduce inflammation in the body and to allow the gut to heal. NB had a severe reaction to sodium sulfites commonly found in wines, and she was a daily red wine drinker. Also, she had a severe reaction to candida. This was consistent with numerous markers in her organic acids test for yeast. NB had moderate reactivity to orange, coconut, vanilla, sweet potato, potato, apple, red and blue food dye, and turmeric. What is interesting is that in this particular case taking turmeric as an anti-inflammatory would actually be increasing inflammation instead of lessening it. NB was instructed to refrain from these foods for 60 days to reduce her inflammation, which decreased the adrenal stress and allowed the gut to heal with the help of some liposome colostrum.

NB had extremely high levels of many environmental toxins, most of which potentially cause cancer. Most of these toxins were coming from her water source. Although she recently moved to the East Coast of Florida, she had spent most of her adult life in New Jersey in close proximity to many industrial facilities. Any one of these numerous chemicals could be enough of a stressor coupled with her BRAC gene to culminate into a subsequent breast cancer. Although there are numerous studies for individual toxins, there are none that evaluate the effect of multiple toxins that stress the same detoxification pathway. Logic, however, dictates that if there are 2, 3, 4, 5, 6 or more of these toxins causing excess body burden there is greater risk for a disease process to occur.

Even though NB had been very particular that she ate only organic food, she did not put the same priority level on her water and air sources. Pure air and water are foundational for good health and are lacking in so many people. Most of us are breathing polluted air and drinking polluted water. You, me, we have to take more personal responsibility for this for ourselves and our families. Moreover, it is our moral responsibility that we make other people aware of this as well. While municipalities may not have the resources to fix the water problem, correction can be made at the supply points, our homes and offices.

NB had 17 different markers for toxic chemicals in her body, anywhere from the low side in the 50th percentile to the high side over the 95th percentile. This means she tested higher than 50 -95% (depending on the percentile) of the thousands of other patients tested. Even though she indicated she ate organic foods only she was still the 50th percentile for glyphosates, which means it was probably coming from the water supply as many of the herbicides wind up in there.

NB had 5 markers in her GPL-Non-Metal Chemical Profile that are known to cause cancer. Again 99% of these could be eliminated by a water filtration system with the NSF/ANSI 401 certification. When body burdens run this high, the body's ability to compensate is overwhelmed. The body uses up its reserve of critical micronutrients, such as glutathione, super oxide dismutase, catalase, B vitamins, magnesium, zinc, selenium, coenzyme Q 10, alpha lipoic acid, and the like. When this happens, the body cannot detoxify the toxins, and cellular dysfunction can occur in multiple tissues. Mothers and fathers wake up. It is no longer a mystery why so many infants and children have learning, behavior disabilities, allergies, and cancer. You have to take charge of the environment at the home and office even before they are born.

NB had a marker in the 100th percentile that is indicative of a gasoline additive. These additives have been demonstrated to cause liver, kidney, and nervous system toxicity and cancer in animals. A water filtration system like the Multipure^{TM} takes this toxin out of the water supply. NB also had a marker for MEP above the 75th percentile. MEP is a marker for phthalates, probably the most widespread in the environment and commonly found in plastics, cosmetics, pharmaceuticals, and bath and beauty products. Diethyl phthalate makes plastics more flexible and appears in many common household products, including food packaging, tools, toothbrushes, toys, aftershave lotions, aspirin, bath   products, cosmetics, detergents, eye shadows, hairsprays, insecticides, mosquito repellants, nail extenders, nail polish, nail polish removers, skin care products, hairstyling products, and auto parts. Adults and children are exposed to phthalates through everyday contact with these products and contact with indoor air and dust. I also recommended that NB use the ActivePure™ air filtration system. Phthalates have been linked to premature birth, reproductive defects, and early onset puberty and additionally linked to cancer, autoimmunity, and organ damage in laboratory tests on rodents. Children's allergies have been linked to exposure to phthalate. Phthalate exposure in pregnant women has changed the anogenital distance in neonatal boys, a change that in rodents exposed to phthalates was associated with genital abnormalities. Use of infant lotion, infant powder, and infant shampoo have been associated with increased infant urine concentrations of phthalate metabolites. Individuals with high values, especially women who want to have children or children who have been exposed, may wish to dramatically reduce their exposures to these substances. Seven European countries have outlawed two major types of the compounds in cosmetics and baby toys. Elimination of MEP, diethyl phthalate, and all phthalates can be accelerated by sauna treatment, by the Hubbard detoxification protocol (known as the Purification Rundown) employing niacin supplementation, or by glutathione (reduced) supplementation (oral, intravenous, transdermal, or precursors such as N-acetyl cysteine [NAC]).

NB had an MHA marker that comes from xylene. Xylene is found not only in common products like paint, lacquers, pesticides, cleaning fluids, fuel and exhaust fumes, but also in perfumes and insect repellants. Xylenes are oxidized in the liver and bowel to glycine before being eliminated by the urine. Xylene increases oxidative stress that can lead to central nervous system depression and even death. These levels were approximately in the 60th percentile.

NB also had a marker for HHPA, a metabolite produced by byproducts of clostridium bacteria, that can inhibit the conversion of dopamine to epinephrine (adrenaline). A high potency probiotic was recommended to combat this. Elevated levels of oxalic acid were detected. Many patients have this sensitivity to oxalates. A list of foods containing high levels of oxalate was given to the patient to help her reduce her intake. I see this sensitivity when patients make a habit of having a green drink with kale, spinach, blueberries, and almonds on a daily basis. I am not saying spinach, kale, blueberries, and almonds are bad for you. I am simply saying that if you are oxalate sensitive, it causes inflammation when you get too much. If you are having reoccurring joint and muscle pain and are having such a drink, you should get tested for it. Her gut dysbiosis could also cause elevated oxalic acids as well. In addition, Vitamin B6, arginine, Vitamin E, chondroitin sulfide, selenium, omega-3 fatty acids, and/or N- acetyl glucosamine supplements may also reduce oxalates and/or their toxicity. See oxalate list below.

- Spinach
- Bran flakes
- Rhubarb
- Beets
- Potato chips
- French fries
- Nuts and nut butters.
- Soy
- Chocolate
- Peanuts
- Tea
- Berries

The Organic Acids Test revealed several other problems that needed some attention. High lactate and pyruvic acid markers were present most probably due to bacterial overgrowth of the GI tract and/or mitochondrial dysfunction. Increasing fermented food intake with a high dosage of probiotics and supplementation of pantothenic acid, lipoic acid, riboflavin, and thiamine that helps with the conversion of the pyruvate acid acetyl-CoA in the mitochondrial energy cycle corrects this condition by improving the microbiome. a

Her elevated succinic acid marker may have indicated a riboflavin and/or coenzyme Q10 deficiency in an enzyme process in the mitochondrial energy cycle that may also be due to gut dysbiosis as levels often decrease after probiotic treatment. Elevated fumaric acid markers also indicated some deficit in the mitochondrial energy function. Recommendations for the mitochondrial function are supplementation of coQ10, NAD (Nicotinamide adenine dinucleotide), l-carnitine, riboflavin, nicotinamide, biotin, and vitamin E. These problems in mitochondrial energy production are significant. If the liver cells cannot produce appropriate mitochondrial energy, an individual cannot detoxify the body.

NB also exhibited high malic acid markers, which indicated a need for niacin and CoQ10 in the mitochondrial energy cycle. She exhibited low VMA (vanylmandelic acid), which means she had a problem with low epinephrine and norepinephrine. This condition can be due to the Clostridium bacteria metabolites or due to a low dietary intake of the amino acids, phenylalanine or tyrosine. Magnesium, B6 or biopterin can be deficient.

NB also exhibited low levels of 5-HIAA (5-hydroxyindoleacetic acid), indicating a lower production of the neurotransmitter serotonin. This lower production can contribute to depression. Supplementation of 5-HTP (5-hydroxytryptophan) helps this deficiency. She also exhibited several markers that could be due to fatty acid oxidation disorders or from an increased consumption of medium chain fatty acids like are found in coconut oil. NB had not been consuming coconut oil or other medium chain fatty acids, so this was thought to be due to a carnitine deficiency. Carnitine is a limiting factor in the use of fatty acids in the mitochondria energy cycle that can be addressed with supplementation with l-carnitine or l-acetyl-carnitine.

Since she had low levels of Vitamin B6, pantothenic acid, and ascorbic acid (Vitamin C), nutritional supplementation was recommended for support of these nutrients. NB also had two markers that indicated she was deficient in intracellular glutathione. Glutathione is critical for multiple detoxification pathways. Replacement can be accomplished with supplementation of reduced glutathione or NAC (N-acetyl cysteine), a precursor to glutathione. I recommended a liquid oral spray that contained both. Glutathione is often deficient in individuals with high environmental body burden because it is used up trying to get rid of the various chemicals from the body.

Her perchlorate, a chemical used in the production of rocket fuel, missiles, fireworks, explosives, fertilizer, and bleach, levels were found to be above the 50th percentile. This compound, often found in water supplies, can disrupt the thyroid's ability to produce hormones. The EPA has also labeled it as a likely carcinogen. A reverse osmosis, better yet a Multipure™ filtration system, will reduce/eliminate this toxin. NB also had a level of TPHP (diphenyl phosphate) above the 70th percentile. TPHP is a metabolite from flame retardant used in plastics, electronic appointment, nail polish, and resins. As an endocrine disruptor, studies have linked it to reproductive and developmental problems. A proper water filtration system, such as the Multipure™, addresses this toxin.

The marker NAPR (N-acetyl propyl cysteine) is a marker for an organic solvent (1-bromopropane) used for metal cleaning, foam gluing, and dry cleaning. Chronic exposure can lead to motor and sensory loss, cognitive loss, and impairment of the central nervous system. NB had levels above the 85th percentile of this environmental toxin in her body. Another marker found in this test is a probable human carcinogen is propylene oxide, a chemical used in the production of plastic and as a food additive, herbicide, insecticide, and fungicide. NB also had a marker for DEP at about the 50% percentile. NB comes from organophosphates that are one of the most toxic substances in the world. This toxin causes overstimulation of the nervous system causing sweating, excess salivation, diarrhea, and abnormal behaviors including autism spectrum disorder.

I made recommendations for her to change her water filtration system to the Multipure™ Aquaperform coupled with the Living Water, which creates hydrogenated, electrolyzed, negatively charged anti-oxidant water, a Multipure™ filter for her shower head, the LaundryPure to remove petrochemicals from her clothing, and the Freshair Everest to remove mold, bacteria, virus, and fine particulates from her breathing space in her home. The combination of these technologies reduced her contamination from water and air as much as is possible.

NB received recommendations for a customize nutritional protocol through our ID life portal taking into account her allergies, genetics, family history, personal history lifestyle, organic acids testing, environmental testing. This formula covered about 80% of her needed nutritional recommendations. In addition, she had recommendations of colloidal silver to help kill her yeast and pathological bacteria, micronized Chlinoptilolite Zeolite for heavy metal chelation, and a combination of NAC, reduce glutathione, acetyl-l-carnitine, L-glutamine, alpha lipoic acid, ascorbic acid oral spray supplementation for additional detoxification, and probiotics. NB also received recommendations for transdermal liposome progesterone and DHEA, prurea murifica to increase her estriol (benign form of estrogen), levels, and a transdermal liposomal

---

product to help support her testosterone levels. Special emphasis was given to support her estrogen detoxification and protection from estrogen-related cancers.

I also made recommendations for some follow up testing for the Nagalese Biofilm test and the CA Discovery Liquid Biopsy Test with another physician who specializes in cancer prevention. The Biofilm test determines the amount of nagalese there is in the body. This is a mucousy material that surrounds cancer tumors as well as chronic infections like MRSA, Lymes, and Candida. A treatment called fatty acid macrophage has been developed to destroy the nagalese so the person's immune system can then deal with it. The CA Discovery Liquid Biopsy Test was developed in a laboratory in Greece and can determine the number of circulating cancer cells in the body. This helps identify the body's ability to handle the cancer. I felt she might benefit from this information.

NB was an example of having some bad genes that were amplified by numerous environmental toxins, most of which were coming through her water supply. Remember that the vast majority of gene variants are actionable, meaning a person can compensate by avoiding certain foods, eating more of specific foods, nutritional supplements, exercise, or stress reduction techniques.

I also recommend the BrainTap^{TM} to my patients for stress reduction.

Case History # 3

KH was a 15-year-old girl who was a friend's granddaughter. She had a history of asthma and multiple allergies, recently developed eczema and was placed on methotrexate, an immunosuppressive medication. She was already on 5 other medications before being placed on methotrexate. This makes for a poor long–term prognosis for this little girl. If she was on 6 medications at age 15, how many do you think she will be by on the time she is 30 if she did not make any changes?

After consultation with KH, her mother, and grandmother, I recommended an autoimmune panel from Great Plains Laboratory. This panel consisted of the Organic Acids Test, GPL-Tox Non-Metal Chemical Profile, Glyphosates, hair analysis for heavy metals and minerals, IgG testing for food allergies, and fatty acids panel. My preferred method of testing food/chemical allergy/sensitivity is with

---

171

MRT (Mediator Release Testing). However, there were budgetary concerns with the family, and I was able to get this particular package of tests discounted somewhat for them. KH had previous skin testing for food allergies but I find this method quite poor overall for determining food allergies as it only assesses IgE type reactions, which are a small minority (5-6%) of the potential food reactivity types.

There is a relationship between certain airborne allergens and specific foods because they contain the same proteins. Reactive foods cause chronic inflammation, which in turn causes a leaky gut by loosening the tight junctions in the single cell epithelial layer in the small intestine. This same inflammation also adversely affects the microbiome. These adverse effects were confirmed by her Organic Acids Test that demonstrated numerous markers for yeast, fungal, and negative bacteria overgrowth. The heavy metal hair analysis revealed elevated levels of aluminum, cadmium, silver, and titanium. Aluminum toxicity is highest in the country in the Tampa Bay, Florida, area where KH is from and in the Miami, Florida, area as well. See Chapter 3: Heavy Metals. KH was advised not to use conventional hair dyes, aluminum cookware or aluminum foil for storage, and no antiperspirants containing aluminum.

The results from the IgG Food Testing revealed severe reactions to Baker's yeast and Brewer's yeast, moderate reaction to Candida Albicans, and mild reactions to gluten, wheat, gliadin (wheat protein), egg white, casein, cow's milk, yogurt, and cheese. I recommended KH be off all sugar, dairy, grains, and eggs for 60 days. This was to reduce gut inflammation and reduce feeding the yeast. Candida thrives on dairy and sugar.

KH demonstrated an 18:1 ratio of omega 6:omega 3 in her Fatty Acid Testing. Levels of 15-20:1 are commonly found in those who eat the standard American diet. An increased severity of asthma symptoms and increased incidence of mental illness, arthritis and heart disease are seen when levels exceed 10:1 ratio of omega 6:omega 3. When levels are below 5:1, the severity of asthma symptoms markedly reduce. Values below 4:1 are associated with good mental health and 70% decrease in cardiovascular disease. The Mediterranean diet produces an approximate ratio of 2.6:1. Suppression of some cancers are seen at a 2.5:1 ratio. The Paleolithic diet (caveman diet) and the traditional Greek diet before 1960 were approximately 1-2:1 ratio. KH was also grossly deficient in Omega 3s. I recommended a liquid supplement of 3 grams/day. It has been my experience that achieving a 1-2:1 omega 6:omega 3 ratio significantly reduces autoimmune responses. This is also true of dramatically increasing Vitamin D levels to 80-100 ng/ mL.

As presented earlier, her Organic Acids Testing demonstrated multiple high yeast/fungal metabolites indicating an overgrowth in the gastrointestinal tract. She also had markers for negative bacteria growth. These changes were consistent with chronic stress/inflammation. KH also demonstrated markers for elevated oxalates. Foods high in oxalates are spinach, beets, soy, chocolate, peanuts, wheat bran, tea, cashews, pecans, almonds, and berries. Oxalic acid is also a byproduct of candida. Excess levels of oxalates need to be reduced because they can interfere with calcium, magnesium, zinc, and other mineral absorption. Typically, I do not see a problem with oxalate intake unless the patient is combining many at one time in smoothie drinks.

KH also had a high succinic acid marker, which is suggestive of low levels of riboflavin and/or CoQ10. Many times, this marker clears after treatment for dysbiosis. Probiotic treatment and supplementation of riboflavin and CoQ10 help resolve this condition. KH also demonstrated two markers that indicated a reduced ability to metabolize the amino acid leucine, which causes problems in the body's ability to make cellular energy. This occurs usually because of some genetic defects in mitochondrial function. Fortunately, this inability is well countered by specific supplementation. Most genetic variations are actionable, meaning action steps inhibit their expression. In this case, supplementation of CoQ10, NAD, l-carnitine, riboflavin, nicotinamide, biotin, and Vitamin E were the action steps.

KH further exhibited low levels of a specific marker indicating lower levels of serotonin, which could lead to depression. This can be corrected by supplementing 5-HTP (5-hydroxytryptophan). She had a marker indicating low B6 levels. The metabolite is involved in a very important pathway associated with several neurodegenerative disorders, including Alzheimer's disease, Parkinson's disease, multiple sclerosis, and Lou Gehrig's disease, ALS (amotrophic laterosclerosis). Tests like this are important in the prevention of neurodegenerative diseases by appropriate supplementation before overt symptoms manifest.

KH had a marker suggestive of neurotoxicity that could be caused by immune overstimulation, excess production of cortisol, and high exposure to phthalates. In her case, all were happening. Fortunately, most of this potential damage can be negated by supplementation of carnitine, melatonin, turmeric (curcumin), garlic, and niacin. Multiple markers were found indicative of nutritional deficiencies of B6, Vitamin C, and glutathione. It should be noted that routine ingestion of acetaminophen (Tylenol) can lead to intracellular glutathione deficiency. Glutathione is one of the three most powerful anti-oxidants our body's produce. The other two are catalase and super oxide dismutase.

The testing revealed this 15-year-old had multiple nutritional deficiencies. This could be due to poor nutritional intake, genetic variations causing poor utilization, or nutritional depletion secondary to heavy environmental toxicity causing specific nutrients to be used up combating the body burden. For most people, as it was with KH, it is a combination of all three factors.

The GPL-Tox Non-Metal Chemical Profile revealed multiple toxins at high levels. See Chapter 12: GPL-TOX: Toxic Non-Metal Chemical Profile for a complete description of the effects of these non-metal chemical. Twelve of the markers were over the 50th percentile, four were over the 75th percentile, and one over the 95th percentile. What this means is that the level of her body burden of these various chemicals was higher than 50 %, 75%, and 95% respectively than all of the other thousands of people tested. This is a perfect example to demonstrate the potential harm environmental toxins can cause an individual. This 15-year-old girl had been placed on 6 medications to mask symptoms caused by her environment. These medications further compromised her body's ability to detoxify. The physician who placed her on these medications never investigated the causation. In fact, he probably never considered that there may be non-drug solutions such as simply removing the poisons.

I tell patients all the time. If you don't want surgery, don't consult with a surgeon. If you don't want an adjustment, don't go see a chiropractor. If you don't want prescription drugs, don't go see your M.D. If you don't want to make changes in your lifestyle, don't come see me.

The first abnormal marker in KH's GPL-Tox was in the 95th percentile for a metabolite that comes from MTBE/EBTE. This exposure most likely comes through ground water contamination. KH had five other markers for environmental toxins over the 75th percentile and several others that were over the 50th percentile. The relative percentile reflects that detection of that particular toxin was greater than that percentage of all people tested which is in the thousands if not tens of thousands. Each of these individual toxins is capable of causing a cascade of inflammation, immune compromise, and mitochondrial damage.

The marker 2,3,4-MHA was in the 90th percentile. KH also had high levels (95th percentile) of HEMA, a byproduct of ethylene chloride, vinyl chloride, and halopropane. Elimination of vinyl chloride can also be accelerated by sauna treatment, niacin supplementation, Vitamin B12 therapy, reduced glutathione, or N-acetyl-cysteine (NAC). She had glyphosates levels near the 95th percentile and three other markers approaching the 75th percentile. PGO (Phenylglyoxylic Acid), DPP, and NABD, a by-product of a chemical, 1, 3 butadiene, made from the processing of petroleum

It is no wonder this 15-year old girl was so sick. What is important to understand is that the vast majority of these environmental toxins cause learning and behavioral developmental problems and cancer. They cause inflammation, immune compromise, hormone and micronutrient depletion, microbiome change, and mitochondrial damage. They cause all of the 7 sequela of stress that were discussed in the introduction. Hopefully, you are getting a better understanding of why ADHD, autism, allergies, autoimmune disease, diabetes, and cancer are on the rise in the population, especially our children.

To summarize, KH was a 15-year-old girl who was taking six different medications, one of which was an immunosuppressant. She had fatigue, asthma, multiple allergies, eczema, chronic reoccurring respiratory and skin related complaints. She was becoming auto-immune. Without intervention, her prognosis was bleak. She was literally being poisoned by the food she ate, the water she drank, and the air she breathed. She had numerous nutritional deficiencies that were not allowing her immune and detoxification systems to function properly. There is no drug made or will ever be made that can replace real, nourishing food and nutritional supplements and pristine drinking water and non-polluted air.

To eliminate her poisoning via her food, air, and water and shore up her nutritional deficiencies to give her a fighting chance, she needed to bullet- proof her home from the many environmental toxins with a new air and water filtration system. I recommended the Multipure™ Aquaperform solid carbon block water filter and the FreshAir Everest with the ActivePure™ technology to remove mold, virus, bacteria, and the many chemicals found in the home from her breathing space. In addition, I recommended the LaundryPure to remove the petro-chemicals from her clothing and keep them from being absorbed through her skin. I also recommended the Living Water to produce hydrogenated, electrolyzed water to help increase her anti-oxidant capabilities. Not only the patient, but the whole family benefited from these recommendations. These are the kind of changes that need to be made for long-term success.

She further needed to eat more organic foods to reduce the glyphosate level in her body. She needed some specific supplementation as indicated from her testing to support detoxification pathways and help kill off the candida, and probiotics to restore her microbiome. In cases like this. I often use 40-100 billion cfus of probiotic daily or a product called Megaspore Biotic™. She was to have no sugar, grains, or dairy for 60 days. I also recommended a liposome colostrum to help heal her leaky gut.

The parents said they could not afford the home water and air system. The entire home system would have cost them about $2,500 and could be made in installments. This amount is less than the amount of money they had spent in out-of-pocket expense for her crisis management sick care the past year, which had no prevention or corrective effect. Since they were not going to get a home unit, I found them a local source where they could purchase quality reverse osmosis water. KH complied with the water and food restrictions for the most part and took the recommended supplements for 60 days. During this time, her skin problems greatly improved, and her breathing was moderately improved, having to use the inhaler much less and no significant asthma episodes. Her energy was better and there were no sick days from school.

Despite this marked improvement, her parents did not follow through with the home protection package recommended and discontinued the additional nutritional supplementation. It usually takes about six months to replenish the body intracellularly for a nutritional deficiency. It is my hope that there will be some future permanent changes in improving the family's water and air supply for KH's sake.

A common problem with patients is lacking the education about what really determines their health and wellness. KH did not get sick because she had a deficiency of the six drugs she was prescribed. She got sick from her environment and her lifestyle, eating the SAD. Many people do not have a good understanding of what makes someone healthy and what makes someone ill. However, it is not uncommon to know someone who said they were feeling well and suddenly had a heart attack or stroke or went in for a routine examination and found they had cancer. Something was going wrong for quite a while for these things to occur. It was just overlooked. In my office, I do wellness assessments to determine nutritional, hormonal, cardiovascular, neurological, and musculoskeletal fitness. I use specific markers for diagnosis. As a result, this book, and other books like it, is necessary to increase awareness.

Case History # 4

SC was a 53-year-old male who was a CEO of a busy and growing construction company. He was 6 feet and weighed 264. He worked out regularly with a personal trainer, but ate and drank too much and didn't get enough sleep. He was diabetic with blood sugars around 250, had a history of ADHD, and possessed the APOE4 gene variant that increases an individual's risk of cardiovascular disease and Alzheimer's. He was taking some nutritional supplements and was on testosterone troche oral dosage. He was highly functional and productive, but he was a walking time bomb because of the elevated blood sugar and APOE4 gene variant that increases the individual's risk for cardiovascular disease and Alzheimer. APOE is responsible for clearing the cholesterol produced by the glial cells from the brain. The APOE4 gene variant is the least efficient in doing this function.

Type 2 diabetes is a killer in more ways than one. If you are diabetic, you have a 400% increased risk for a heart attack or stroke, regardless of any other risk factors. The diabetic individual may appear to be doing okay and then suddenly overnight his/her body breaks down. Type 2 diabetes is preventable, treatable, and reversible. You just have to be willing to change some things in your lifestyle and take some supplements for a while. Individuals often think they have more time. The time is now to take action steps to stop or reverse diabetes.

Type 2 diabetes, generally speaking, is caused by insulin resistance for the most part. However, as time goes by these individuals often become insulin insufficient necessitating exogenous insulin treatment. The pancreatic beta cells fail to produce adequate insulin over time, and insulin injections become necessary. The slender type II diabetic is often insulin deficient. This accounts for about 20% of total diabetes type II. Insulin insufficiency often responds well to supplementation of the Ayurvedic herb, gynema. Type I diabetics have auto-immune damage to the pancreatic beta cells.

I asked SC to fill out a general history, thyroflex questionnaire, and system survey questionnaire. Several years of prior medical records were reviewed as well. The thyroflex questionnaire focuses on thyroid, adrenal, and melatonin problems. The system survey form consists of 200 questions broken down into several categories. The system survey form revealed 23% of his complaints were related to hormone imbalance/deficiencies, 21% to liver- gallbladder dysfunction, 18% to digestive dysfunction, and 13% to blood sugar dysregulation. These four systems accounted for 75% of his complaints. It should be kept in mind that insulin is a master hormone and when there is an imbalance here the influences are felt in multiple systems. The system survey questionnaire has a potential 1000 points for a perfect score. SC scored 200. That would be 20% or an F in school. No one wants an F for a wellness/health score. The scores correspond to SC's top 5 complaints: sleeping problems, blood sugar fluctuation problems causing carbohydrate cravings, clouded thought processes, frequent tiredness, and easily and often distracted.

In order to get a better understanding of what was going on with SC, I recommended assessing his thyroid and sex hormones, a cardio-metabolic blood profile, an Organic Acids Test, GPL-Tox Non-Metal Chemical Profile, Glyphosate test, and PLA2 test. The last four tests can all be done through one urinalysis. The thyroflex testing for measuring intracellular T3 levels was done in the office. I also conducted testing with the Maxpulse™, which evaluates four cardiovascular functions and heart rate variability.

The heart rate variability demonstrated low hormonal function, and one of the cardiovascular indicators demonstrated arterial elasticity at a suboptimal level. His resting heart rate was 55, a pulse rate you might expect for a serious runner or cross-fit athlete but he was neither. This lower heart rate was suggestive of a hypothyroid function, which was confirmed by the thyroflex testing. His thyroflex score using the speed of his brachioradialis reflex was over 200 milliseconds with ideal readings for the thyroid being between 50-100 milliseconds. Marginal readings for thyroid function are between 100-120 milliseconds. Please refer to the 2nd Edition of *13 Secrets to Optimal Aging: How Your Hormones Can Help You Achieve a Better Quality of Life and Longevity* to get more details on thyroflex testing for thyroid function.

Saliva hormone testing revealed his free testosterone levels were above the maximum testing level of 928.9 pg/milliliter. His estradiol and estrone levels were both elevated as well. It is common for aging men to convert more testosterone and estrogen. He needed his current testosterone dosage reduced slightly. and he certainly needed his estrogen levels reduced and needed estrogen detoxification protection as well. Elevated estrogen levels in the aging male are associated with increased prostate and breast cancer and cardiovascular risk. His DHEA and cortisol levels were low, indicating adrenal cortex hypofunction or fatigue. Low DHEA and cortisol also causes diminished secretory IgA, which is the protective mucous membrane covering the lining of the small intestine, resulting in a leaky gut, hyperpermeability of the protective epithelial layer of cells in the small intestine. A follow-up MRT (Mediator Release Test) was recommended to assess food/chemical allergies/sensitivities contributing to inflammation in his gut.

SC's lipid profile was the following: 264 total cholesterol, 448 triglycerides, with only a 34 for HDL. This is a cholesterol/HDLC ratio of 7.8. Optimal is under 3. His triglycerides/HDLC ratio was 13, optimal is below 2. The triglycerides/HDL ratio is a better predictor for cardiovascular risk than the total cholesterol/HDL according to studies from Framingham, the largest on-going study on cardiovascular risks. His HgA1c was 8.4. A level under 5.7 is considered normal. His Vitamin D 25-OH total was 37 ng/mL. Ideal levels are in the upper quartile, 80-100 ng/mL. His LDLs sub-fractions also put him at a high risk for cardiovascular disease/event. When a physician sees this kind of test information, it is time to have a heart-to-heart with the patient. SC had multiple risk factors for a cardiovascular event and Alzheimer's. It is part of the physician's job to help patients be accountable for his/her own health.

The Organic Acids Test is a nutritional, metabolic profile encompassing yeast/fungal markers, bacteria markers, oxalate metabolites, mitochondrial markers, neurotransmitter markers, folate metabolism, ketone and fatty acid oxidation markers, vitamins, amino acids, and mineral nutritional markers. SC had 12 different markers for yeast/fungal and bacteria overgrowth. This was a confirmation of the 6th sequela of stress, leaky gut and microbiome change. SC also had 4 different markers for mitochondrial energy production problems, the 7th sequela of stress. SC had a marker that indicated a lower production of the neurotransmitter, norepinephrine, and/or the hormone, adrenaline. SC also exhibited a marker indicating his serotonin levels were low. Serotonin is a calming neurotransmitter that helps the brain synchronize left and right brain information. SC also had a marker for neurotoxicity that could be negated by taking a supplement of niacin, B3. Niacin also helps elevate HDL, something SC needed. SC also exhibited markers indicating he was using more fatty acids for energy, but was having problems transporting them into the mitochondria due to a carnitine deficiency. Supplementation of l-carnitine or acetyl l-carnitine will help correct this problem. Other nutritional markers indicated Vitamin B12, Vitamin C, and glutathione deficiencies. All of these nutrients are critical for numerous body functions. Supplementation of these nutrients was part of his recommendations.

The environmental testing revealed 4 markers to be significantly elevated. The first marker was for some gasoline additives used to improve octane. The most likely exposure is through ground water. These compounds have been demonstrated to cause liver, kidney, and central nervous system toxicity, peripheral nerve toxicity (neuropathy), and cancer in animals. The chemicals excretion half-life of this toxin is 10-28 hours which means he had been poisoned recently and probably on a regular basis through his tap water. Using a water filter with the new NSF/ANSI 401 rating removes 99% of this from his drinking water. Use of a sauna with near and infra-red light and glutathione or N-acetylcysteine MAC supplementation accelerates the detoxification of these compounds from the body.

Another chemical found in concentrations over the 75th percentile was styrene. He had a body burden of HEMA at the 100th percentile. Prevention of this contamination can be secured with the use of a water filtration system with the NSF/ANSI 401 rating. Elimination of these toxins can be accelerated through the use of sauna or glutathione or NAC supplementation. Another chemical found in concentrations at the 100th percentile was 1-bromo-propane. This exposure may have occurred at a construction site, but also from dry-cleaning of his Hawaiian-type shirt that he wore daily without an undershirt. This toxicity may have come from transdermal exposure from the dry-cleaning. I advised him to wear and undershirt laundered with the LaundryPure to avoid further transdermal exposure to this chemical. The fourth chemical in concentrations near the 75th percentile was NAHP. See Chapter 12: GPL-TOX: Toxic Non-Metal Chemical Profile
for more information about these chemicals.

As I wrote earlier, this patient was a walking time bomb. He needed assistance on many levels to reduce his risk for a cardiovascular event and reduce the body burden of multiple toxins, which were all carcinogenic. The two priorities I had were to stop the environmental poisoning and to significantly reduce his blood sugar levels. Recommendations were made for him to reduce his environmental poisoning from the air and particularly his water with a Multipure™ water filtration system coupled with the Living Water for electrolyzed reduced water and LaundryPure and an air filtration system with the ActivePure™ technology. The second priority was specific nutritional support that included the herb genema, bitter lemon, chromium nicotinamide (chromate), and alpha lipoic acid. Pharmaceutical grade genema increases the pancreatic beta cell production of insulin.

My nutritional recommendations were part of a personalized custom-made nutritional protocol that encompassed some 55-60 different nutrients. These recommendations came from evaluating his family history, personal history, lifestyle, test results, and experience with similar conditions in other patients. The nutraceuticals were to help support blood sugar regulation, adrenal and thyroid functions, and cardiovascular system. SC was also given bioidentical hormone supplement recommendations of transdermal liposomal pregnenolone and DHEA and a transdermal to increase testosterone. I recommended SC quit taking his oral testosterone dosing due to potential liver stress.

One of the things I talked to SC about was getting to bed at the same time (an earlier time) every night and getting up at the same time every day. He had a two- to three-hour variance in his going to bed and getting up times. Sleeping from 10 PM to 2 AM is critical for healing. This is when the parasympathetic nervous system (digestion and healing) is most active. This is optimum time for the body to detoxify and rejuvenate. To help SC to accomplish this new sleeping pattern, I recommended SC use a technology called BrainTap^{TM} on a regular basis. There are over 700 different programs available on BrainTap^{TM} that can be used for a wide variety of purposes. Generally, using it is great for stress reduction and behavior modification. Most of the 15-20 minute programs are designed to help inhibit the sympathetic nervous system (fight/flight) response and encourage the parasympathetic nervous system and calming neurotransmitters GABA and serotonin. The headset uses three different audio technologies and two light technologies. I've had a good response with several type II diabetics in reducing their blood sugars with the BrainTap^{TM}. Since most people feel stressed-out these days, they produce high amounts of adrenaline and cortisol. Cortisol, also known as glucosteroid, increases sugar production. The more cortisol that is produced the more sugar is produced. The BrainTap^{TM} reduces the fight/flight response stress response, which decreases the cortisol and, thereby, decreases the blood sugars.

SC's blood sugar levels dropped 100 points within 30 days, averaging between the130s to 150s. This was despite less than full compliance with recommendations. Further improvements came after SC stopped eating the reactive foods that were demonstrated in the MRT. Another 60 days saw a 25-pound weight loss and further reduction of his blood sugars to the 90s to 100s. His HgA1c dropped to 6.0. Normal is considered below 5.7. His HDL levels increased to 48 and his tryglcerides dropped to 165. His trigyceride/HDLC ratio went from 13 to 3.4. Ideal is < 2. He was almost there.

Glossary

1-Bromopropane (1-BP)—an organic solvent, used for metal cleaning, foam gluing, and dry cleaning, that is a neurotoxin as well as a reproductive toxin

1,3 Butadiene—a chemical made from the processing of petroleum. It is often a colorless gas with a mild gasoline-like odor. Most of it is used in the production of synthetic rubber. It is a known carcinogen and has been linked to increased risk of cardiovascular disease.

2, 4-Dicholorophenoxyacetic (2,4-D)—a very common herbicide. Exposure to 2, 4-D via skin or oral ingestion is associated with neuritis, weakness, nausea, abdominal pain, headache, dizziness, peripheral neuropathy, stupor, seizures, brain damage, and impaired reflexes. It is also a known endocrine disruptor that can block hormone distribution and cause glandular breakdown.

4-nonylphenol—substance contained in industrial detergents that is an endocrine disruptor and mimics estrogen.

ACE inhibitor—a type of blood pressure medication

Acrylamide—used in many industrial processes such as plastics, food packaging, cosmetics, nail polish, dyes, and treatment of drinking water. High levels of acrylamide can elevate a patient's risk of cancer and cause neurological damage.

Acrylonitrile—a colorless, odorless carcinogen found in acrylics and cigarettes that is negated by glutathione

ActivePure™—a patented air purification technology that is NASA approved and used in the space station

ADHD—attention deficit hyperactivity disorder

Alzheimer's disease—the most common type of dementia denoted by amyloid beta and Tau protein plaquing

Allopathic—the practice of using drugs, radiation, and surgery for treatment

Aluminum—an abundant mineral on the planet that permeates air, food, and water supplies and bio-accumulating causing neurotoxicity. It is a preservative in many vaccines.

Antimony—a metal found in the earth's crust. It can be toxic and cumulative.

Aquaporin—a positively charged water channel inside the cell that allows one molecule of water in at a time as long as the water is negatively charged as nature intended.

Arabinogalactans—a dietary fiber that aids immune health

Autism—a condition from multiple causes including genetic variances, nutritional deficiencies, EMFs, and environmental toxins that cause learning, social, and behavioral challenges.

Auto-immune disease—when the body makes antibodies against itself, thought to be due to cellular mimicry, a condition wherein the antibody formed against a foreign protein attacks the tissues of an individual because of the similarity in structure. An over-sensitized immune system.

Autonomic imbalance—a disruption of the body's ability to appropriately shift back and forth between the two systems – sympathetic (fight/flight) and parasympathetic (digestion and sleep). Locked into the fight/flight usually.

Benzene—a widespread environmental organic solvent that is a by-product of all sources of combustion, including cigarette smoke and numerous industrial processes. It is released as a vapor from synthetic materials. Extremely toxic, it is mutagenic and carcinogenic.

Boswelia—an anti-inflammatory herb used in Ayurvedic medicine

BPA (Bisphenol A)—contained in some plastics and an endocrine disruptor linked to diabetes and hypothyroidism and obesity.

BRAC—gene variants that increase an individual's risk for breast, uterine, or ovarian cancers.

Braverman—questionnaires to help determine the dominant neurotransmitter in an individual as well as levels of deficiencies

Bromine—a halide that is added to some breads and occurs on many plastic products that is toxic and can have adverse effects on the thyroid.

Cadmium—a naturally occurring toxic heavy metal

Calcium channel blocker —a type of blood pressure medication

Catalase—one of the most powerful endogenous anti-oxidants that is important in protecting against environmental toxins

CDC (Center for Disease Control and Prevention)—federal agency acting under Department of Health and Human Services. Its impartiality has been questioned more than once, such as the time that it redefined several smaller diseases as AIDS in order to bolster the number of cases and assure its funding and when reporting that all vaccines are safe.

Chloride——a toxic substance commonly added to water to kill bacteria

Chlorinated pesticides—bioaccumulates in brain and fat and DDT is the best example

Colostrum—a substance produced in the first milk of mammals that has immune enhancing results and helps leaky gut.

Cortisol—a hormone produced by the adrenal cortex that facilitates glucose production in response to a stressor—mechanical, chemical, or emotional

Cytokines—proteins produced by cells of the immune system causing inflammation

DHEA—an anabolic hormone produced by the adrenal cortex that is important in brain health, bone density, muscle strength, and immune response.

Diabetes—a condition in which blood sugar (glucose) levels are too high that is caused by insulin resistance or insulin insufficiency causing the production of AGEs (advanced glycation end-products) that damage the blood vessels, brain, and other tissues.

EMFs—electromagnetic frequencies originating from certain machinery, large electrical wires, computers, cell towers, cell phones, and WI-FI that increases risk for certain cancers, infertility, blood brain barrier permeability, ADHD, autism spectrum, Alzheimer's disease

ERW—electrolyzed water that goes through an electrolysis process causing it to release hydrogen gas and become negatively charged as demonstrated by an ORP meter. Mimics naturally reduced water and is anti-oxidant

EPA—the Environmental Protection Agency

Eosinophilic—involving an increased production of eosinophils, a type of white blood cell that is involved with allergic reactions

Ethylene Oxide—used in agrochemicals detergents, pharmaceuticals, personal care products, and a sterilizing agent on rubber, plastics, and electronics that has been reported as a carcinogen. It detoxifies with glutathione.

Fibrinolysis— anti-clotting function in the blood

Fluoride—a toxic substance that is often added to toothpaste and mouthwash and can occur in well and ground water.

FreshAir Everest—an air purification system that cleans 3,000 square feet and features the NASA approved ActivePure™ technology

Glutathione—one of the most powerful endogenous antioxidants important in the detoxification of many environmental toxins

Glycocalyx—a meshwork connected to the endothelium that acts like a Teflon-coating to protect the blood vessels from plaquing

Glyphosate—an herbicide in Round-Up™ produced by Monsanto that causes multiple health issues and is commonly found in food and water sources

GMO—genetically modified foods that have contributed to increased allergies and multiple other illnesses. While increasing yields, the crops have less nutritional value than traditional crops.

GPL-Tox Non-Metal Profile— by Great Plains Labs, a comprehensive assessment of environmental toxins other than heavy metals provided

Hashimoto's disease—an auto-immune form of hypothyroidism— 80 % of adults are hypothyroid with 20% of these having Hashimoto's. The condition is worsened by environmental triggers.

Histamine—a substance produced in a localized immune response that causes inflammation. A person can produce histamines in response to certain foods. It is a neurotransmitter.

HRV (heart rate variability)—the difference between the variation in timing between heart beats

Hypospadias—when the urethra does not exit at the end of the penis, but somewhere along the shaft.

IgA—a type of allergic reaction

IgE—a fast acting type of allergic reaction that can be severe and life-threatening like a peanut allergy that closes off the airway

IgG—a type of delayed allergic reaction causing symptoms that can appear 24-72 hours after ingestion of offending food(s)

IgM —another type of allergic reaction

Inflammation—a response the body has to a stressor whether mechanical, chemical, or emotional

Insulin resistance—when there is adequate inulin production but the insulin cell receptor is unable to get glucose through the cell membrane inside the cell to fuel the mitochondria

Iodine—an essential mineral that is commonly deficient and found primarily in sea vegetation

KSCA (Kid-Safe Chemical Act)—legislation that forced companies to prove a product was safe before they brought it to market.

LaundryPure—a device that connects to the washing machine that facilitates the cleaning of clothes without detergent or fabric softener by acidifying the water and producing hydrogen peroxide

Leaky gut—when food and microbes can pass through the tight junctions of the small intestine

Levothyroxin—a generic medication for Synthroid providing a synthetic form of T4

L-glutamine—an essential amino-acid that helps intestinal health

Liposome—the process involving the envelopment of a nutrient or hormone in phosphatidyl choline, a naturally occurring fat in the cell membrane, making it more bio-available to pass through the cell membrane

Living Water—an electrolyzed water system that I recommend to my patients because it provides antioxidant water at a reasonable cost.

Mercury —a neurotoxic substance found commonly in older dental amalgams, large predatory fish, high fructose corn syrup, and some vaccines

Micronutrient test—a blood panel that measures intracellular levels of 35 different vitamins, minerals, and anti-oxidants

mRNA—messenger RNA that is responsible for carrying the duplication information for the mitochondria

MRT—a highly reliable and accurate test that measures the relative inflammatory reactivity to specific foods and chemicals

MTBE (methyl tertiary-butyl ether)—a flammable, colorless toxic liquid used as a gasoline additive that dissolves easily in water and has been found in many water sources. It does not accumulate in the body

Multipure aquaperfom—a type of sold carbon block water filtration system with the 401 Emerging Compounds Certification from NSF that I recommend to my patients

Mycotoxins —bad metabolites from mold that can have a negative impact on health

NRW (naturally reduced water)—water that comes from the healing waters of the planet and some deep well water. It is negatively charged when tested with an ORP meter and contains hydrogen gas that donates an electron to free radicals; an anti-oxidant water

NSF—an international, independent, accrediting organization that tests audits, and certifies products and systems

Obesity—body fat of over 30 % in men and 35% in women

Obesogens—environmental chemicals that cause an individual to have increased body fat

Organic Acid Test —a urinalysis test that evaluates metabolic and detoxification pathways, neurotransmitters, nutritional deficiencies, and mitochondrial energy capabilities

Organophosphates—one of the most toxic groups of substances are often used as biochemical weapons and terrorist agents as well as in pesticides. They are inhibitors of cholinesterase enzymes that lead to overstimulation and abnormal behavior, including aggression and depression. Children exposed to these chemicals have more than twice the risk of developing pervasive developmental disorder (PDD) and autism spectrum disorder.

ORP—oxidation reduction potential or the ability to give up an electron to bind to a free radical

Parabens—additive in personal care products that is an endocrine disruptor

Parasympathetic Nervous System—the part of the autonomic nervous system that controls digestion and sleep

Parkinson's disease—a neurodegenerative disease involving a loss of dopamine in the substantia nigra leading to increased loss of motor control

PCB (Polychlorinated Biphenyls)—found in lubricants and coolants in past. Toxicity is still common even though banned in 1979.

Perchlorate—used in the production of rocket fuel, missiles, fireworks, flares, explosives, fertilizers, and bleach. It has been found in some water supplies and contaminates many food sources. It can disrupt the thyroid's ability to produce hormones. The EPA has also labeled perchlorate a likely human carcinogen.

$PM_{2.5}$—fine particulates in the air that are less that are $< .25$ microns in size, including all bacteria, virus, mold. It is not cleared by HEPA filters and can go through blood-brain barrier.

PM_{10}—larger particulates in the air cleaned by HEPA filters

ppb—parts per billion

ppm—parts per million

Pregnenolone Steal—when the majority of the hormone production is being shunted to making cortisol and the production of other hormones like DHEA and testosterone are lowered

Prion diseases—neurodegenerative diseases in the brain denoted by misfolded proteins

Propylene Oxide—used in the production of plastics and as a fumigant, to make polyester resins for textile and construction industries, and in the preparation of lubricants, surfactants, and oil demulsifiers. It has also been used as a food additive, an herbicide, a microbicide, an insecticide, a fungicide, and a miticide. Propylene oxide is a probable human carcinogen.

Prostaglandins—a group of fatty acid compounds that have hormone-like effects including uterine contractions

Pthalates—component in plastics that make them soft and pliable. Most concentrated pollutant in our bodies and an endocrine disruptor.

Pyrethrins—widely used in insecticides. Exposure during pregnancy doubles the likelihood of autism. They may affect neurological development, disrupt hormones, induce cancer, and suppress the immune system.

Selenium—an essential mineral needed to convert T4 to T3

Sequela—resulting from

SIBO—small intestine overgrowth tested with an inhalation test

Solanine—an alkaloid toxin that can be found in uncooked potatoes, tomatoes, and eggplant

Styrene—used in the manufacturing of plastics and building materials that is found in car exhaust fumes. Polystyrene and its copolymers are commonly used as food-packaging materials. It adversely impacts the central nervous system, causes concentration problems, muscle weakness, tiredness and nausea, and irritates the mucous membranes of the eyes, nose, and throat.

Superoxide dismutase—one of the most powerful endogenous anti-oxidants that helps protect the cell membranes and mitochondria

Sympathetic Nervous System—the fight/flight or stress response part of the nervous system.

Synthroid—a commonly prescribed medication for hypothyroidism providing a synthetic form of T4.

Testosterone—an androgenic hormone produced by the testicles in men and adrenal cortex in women

Thermosil—methyl mercury contained in some vaccines

Tiglylglycine (TG)—a marker for mitochondrial dysfunction. Mutations of mitochondria DNA may result from exposure to toxic chemicals, infections, inflammation, and nutritional deficiencies.

Thyroflex—a FDC cleared device that measures intracellular T3 levels through reflexometry of the brachioradialis muscle with an accuracy of 98.5 %.

Tight junctions—the connections between the single cell endothelial lining of the blood vessels in the brain and the single cell epithelium layer lining the small intestine

Triclosan—antiseptic that bioaccumulates in the body causing thyroid dysfunction

TSH (thyroid stimulating hormone)—produced by the pituitary gland. It stimulates the thyroid to produce T4.

Turmeric—an herbal plant commonly used as seasoning in eastern Indian food

Vinyl Chloride—an intermediate in the synthesis of several commercial chemicals, including polyvinyl chloride (PVC). Exposure to vinyl chloride may cause central nervous system depression, nausea, headache, dizziness, liver damage, degenerative bone changes, thrombocytopenia, enlargement of the spleen, and death.

WHO—World Health Organization

Xenoestogens—chemicals that mimic the effect of estrogen in the body. A common problem today with excess body burden increasing the risk for estrogen–related cancers, such as prostate, breast, uterine, ovarian.

Xylenes (dimethylbenzenes)—solvents found not only in common products such as paints, lacquers, pesticides, cleaning fluids, fuel and exhaust fumes, but also in perfumes and insect repellents. High exposures to xylene create an increase in oxidative stress, causing symptoms such as nausea, vomiting, dizziness, central nervous system depression, and death.

Other books by Dr. Kelly Miller

13 Secrets to Optimal Health: How Your Hormones Can Help You Achieve a Better Quality of Life and Longevity, 2nd edition

Micronutrient Testing: How to Find What Vitamins, Minerals, and Antioxidants You Need., 2nd edition

Saving Your Brain: Causes, Prevention, and Reversal of Dementia/Alzheimer's (in press)

Made in the USA
Las Vegas, NV
13 May 2021